African American Hospitals
in North Carolina

ALSO BY PHOEBE ANN POLLITT
AND FROM MCFARLAND

*African American and Cherokee Nurses in Appalachia:
A History, 1900–1965*

African American Hospitals in North Carolina
39 Institutional Histories, 1880–1967

PHOEBE ANN POLLITT

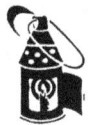

McFarland & Company, Inc., Publishers
Jefferson, North Carolina

LIBRARY OF CONGRESS CATALOGUING-IN-PUBLICATION DATA

Names: Pollitt, Phoebe, author.
Title: African American hospitals in North Carolina : 39 institutional histories, 1880–1967 / Phoebe Ann Pollitt.
Description: Jefferson, North Carolina : McFarland & Company, Inc., Publishers, 2017. | Includes bibliographical references and index.
Identifiers: LCCN 2017033537 | ISBN 9781476667249 (softcover : acid free paper) ∞
Subjects: LCSH: African Americans—Hospitals—North Carolina—History—19th century. | African Americans—Hospitals—North Carolina—History—20th century. | African Americans in medicine. | Equality—Health aspects. | African Americans—Medical care.
Classification: LCC RA981.A45 P65 2017 | DDC 362.1109756—dc23
LC record available at https://lccn.loc.gov/2017033537

BRITISH LIBRARY CATALOGUING DATA ARE AVAILABLE

ISBN (print) 978-1-4766-6724-9
ISBN (ebook) 978-1-4766-3084-7

© 2017 Phoebe Ann Pollitt. All rights reserved

No part of this book may be reproduced or transmitted in any form or by any means, electronic or mechanical, including photocopying or recording, or by any information storage and retrieval system, without permission in writing from the publisher.

Front cover image: Quality Hill Sanatorium, Monroe, North Carolina, ca. 1912 (courtesy North Carolina Department of Archives and History)

Printed in the United States of America

McFarland & Company, Inc., Publishers
 Box 611, Jefferson, North Carolina 28640
  www.mcfarlandpub.com

For Doug, Andy, Betty, Whitley,
Oscar, Winston, Olivia, Bruce,
Danny, Susy, Linda and Bill.
You all have enriched my life
beyond measure.

One horrifying incident:
On the pleasant evening of December 6, 1950, Matthew Avery, a 24-year-old World War II veteran and college student, was involved in a serious car accident near Mebane, North Carolina. He suffered a broken skull, cheekbone, jaw, arm, and leg. An ambulance took Avery to nearby Alamance General Hospital, but the hospital had no room for him. He was then transferred to Duke Hospital, in Durham, North Carolina, about an hour away. Again, he was turned away for lack of room. He was then transferred across town to Lincoln Hospital where he died about an hour after he was admitted. It will never be known if he died from the injuries he sustained in the accident or if he died because he was African American.

—"Hospital refuses," 1950, December 9, *Durham Carolina Times*, p. 1

Acknowledgments

Meg Ruggiero and Michelle Kizer have greatly improved this book through careful reading, knowledge of grammar and punctuation, and helpful suggestions to increase clarity in my writing. Thanks to you both. Rachel Colby was invaluable in creating the map and assisting with the technical aspects of the photographs that appear in the book.

Table of Contents

Acknowledgments   vii

Part I: Historical Overview of Segregated Hospital Care in North Carolina   1

A Brief Review of the Professional Literature   3
A Brief History of Hospitals in North Carolina Through 1900   6
The Establishment of Early General Hospitals, 1876–1900   10
The Founding of African American Hospitals   10
Military and Veteran's Administration (VA) Hospitals   17
Nursing Education   18
Legal Segregation, Social Conditions and Medical Racism   20
20th-Century Statistics Documenting Health Disparities   23
Disparities in Hospital Beds by Race in the Mid–20th Century   24
The Duke Endowment   25
The Rosenwald Fund   26
The North Carolina Medical Care Commission   27
The Hospital Survey and Construction Act/Hill-Burton Act   29
Lawsuits to End Hospital Segregation   30
Conclusion   35

Part II: The Health Care Facilities   37

Raleigh, Wake County   37
Charlotte, Mecklenburg County   56
Southern Pines, Moore County   65
Durham, Durham County   70
Winston-Salem, Forsyth County   76
Wilson, Wilson County   86
Asheville, Buncombe County   92

Henderson, Vance County 101
Monroe, Union County 107
Greensboro, Guilford County 110
Oxford, Granville County 117
Smithfield, Johnston County 121
Gastonia, Gaston County 125
Wilmington, New Hanover County 128
Mount Olive, Wayne County 135
Greenville, Pitt County 136
Statesville, Iredell County 138
Laurinburg, Scotland County 140
New Bern, Craven County 142
Tarboro, Edgecombe County 147
Fayetteville, Cumberland County 150
Conclusion 154

Appendix I: Publicly Supported Specialty Hospitals for African Americans in North Carolina 159

Goldsboro, Wayne County 160
Sanatorium, Hoke County 164

Appendix II: Timeline of Significant Events Related to African American Hospitals in North Carolina, 1865–1965 169

Appendix III: 42 Public and Private African American Hospitals in North Carolina, 1880–1967 172

References 175

Index 195

PART I

Historical Overview of Segregated Hospital Care in North Carolina

Overall life expectancy for residents in the United States increased from 47 years in 1900 to 70 years by 1965 (Life expectancy, 1998). The primary explanations for this rise have been debated for half a century. Dr. Thomas McKeown (1979) led the argument that rising standards of living due to economic growth and better nutrition have been the key factors in increased longevity. Colgrove (2002), Grundy (2004) and others find advances in pharmacology, surgical techniques, care in modern hospitals and immunizations have played at least as important a role in lengthening people's lives as factors identified by McKeown. Both advocates and detractors of the "McKeown Thesis" agree that having access to medical, surgical, pharmacological and nursing care inside a modern hospital is advantageous to health and longevity.

As the medical profession developed in the late 19th and early 20th centuries, white Americans experienced a revolution of life-saving opportunities. New drugs and technologies, the standardization of training for doctors and nurses, readily available modern hospitals, and advances in the science and practice of medicine and nursing led to better and longer lives. These wonders of modern medicine and public health did not come evenly to all Americans. Those with less money and power got less access to new medicines and treatments, and African Americans faced extraordinary difficulty in receiving any health care at all. Often turned away from hospitals and deprived of doctors, nurses, clinics, and medicine, people of color suffered and died unnecessarily in great numbers.

African Americans faced serious social and health inequities in

Part I—Historical Overview

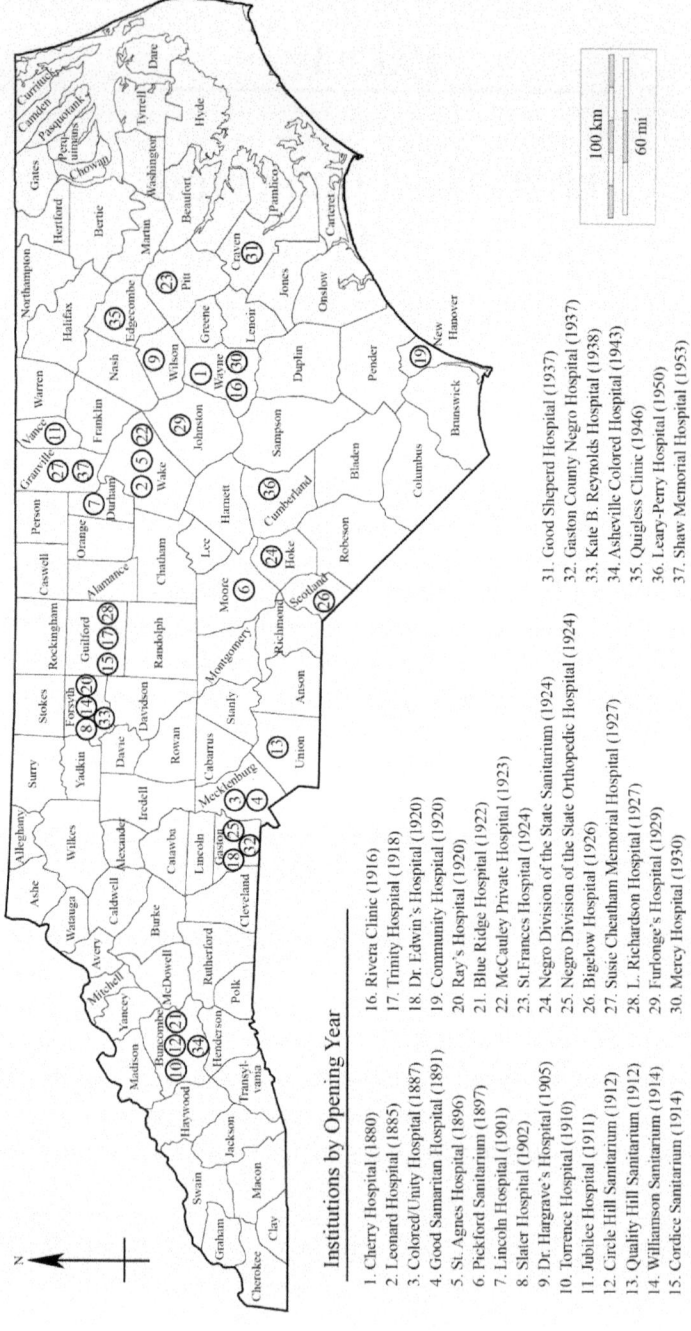

African American Health Care Institutions in North Carolina, 1880–1965.

Institutions by Opening Year

1. Cherry Hospital (1880)
2. Leonard Hospital (1885)
3. Colored/Unity Hospital (1887)
4. Good Samaritan Hospital (1891)
5. St. Agnes Hospital (1896)
6. Pickford Sanitarium (1897)
7. Lincoln Hospital (1901)
8. Slater Hospital (1902)
9. Dr. Hargrave's Hospital (1905)
10. Torrence Hospital (1910)
11. Jubilee Hospital (1911)
12. Circle Hill Sanitarium (1912)
13. Quality Hill Sanitarium (1912)
14. Williamson Sanitarium (1914)
15. Cordice Sanitarium (1914)
16. Rivera Clinic (1916)
17. Trinity Hospital (1918)
18. Dr. Edwin's Hospital (1920)
19. Community Hospital (1920)
20. Ray's Hospital (1920)
21. Blue Ridge Hospital (1922)
22. McCauley Private Hospital (1923)
23. St. Frances Hospital (1924)
24. Negro Division of the State Sanitarium (1924)
25. Negro Division of the State Orthopedic Hospital (1924)
26. Bigelow Hospital (1926)
27. Susie Cheatham Memorial Hospital (1927)
28. L. Richardson Hospital (1927)
29. Furlonge's Hospital (1929)
30. Mercy Hospital (1930)
31. Good Sheperd Hospital (1937)
32. Gaston County Negro Hospital (1937)
33. Kate B. Reynolds Hospital (1938)
34. Asheville Colored Hospital (1943)
35. Quigless Clinic (1946)
36. Leary-Perry Hospital (1950)
37. Shaw Memorial Hospital (1953)

the late 19th and 20th centuries in North Carolina. Grinding poverty, substandard housing, insufficient heat, poor ventilation, inadequate diet, unregulated work environments, untreated water and sewage, overwork, and lack of access to medical care contributed to multiple health problems. These ranged from malnutrition to infectious diseases, including leading causes of morbidity and mortality such as tuberculosis, typhoid, pneumonia, diphtheria, pellagra, and hookworm. Most of the conditions that caused poor health in African Americans in North Carolina were created by Jim Crow/apartheid policies as well as by the pervasively racist society in which they lived. Responding to these dire conditions, scores of African American physicians, nurses and other health professionals—along with a few white allies—built hospitals, sanitariums, and clinics to serve those the white-power structure had abandoned (Gamble, 1989).

The African American struggle for equality has been fought on many fronts, including long battles for citizenship rights, economic opportunity, quality education, and social equality. These aspects of the long Civil Rights Movement are of great historical importance and have received significant scholarly attention. The struggle for fair and equitable health care, however, is largely overlooked. It is the story of a deadly inequality that has much to tell present Americans about the depth and persistence of racial discrimination under both the *de jure* segregation of the past and *de facto* discrimination that continues into the 21st century. It is also a story about African American agency illustrated by the actions of heroic individuals and communities to build and staff African American hospitals. These and other brave individuals later worked to integrate modern medical facilities, providing lifesaving care to all North Carolinians regardless of race.

This book illuminates largely unheralded people and institutions who worked diligently to save lives, improve health, and train others in health professions under almost impossible circumstances. Most of their names and deeds are forgotten, but their courage and dedication deserve recognition. In addition, a deeper understanding of the effects racist policies and laws have had on the health care system may help us create a more equitable and compassionate future.

A Brief Review of the Professional Literature

North Carolina was home to at least 39 private and three public hospitals, sanatoria, and clinics that served African Americans during the decades of legal racial segregation from 1880 to 1965, known as the Jim Crow era. About half of these institutions were built and owned by African American physicians, while the others were joint efforts in which African Americans worked with white allies, philanthropists, religious denominations, and/or government entities to establish hospitals. Most of these hospitals, sanatoria, and clinics have received scant attention in the professional literature. Four such hospitals—Lincoln Hospital, Kate B. Reynolds Hospital, St. Agnes Hospital, Slater Hospital—were the subject of articles in the *Journal of the National Medical Association* (JNMA), the journal produced the organization of African American physicians who were banned from the American Medical Association because of their race. Others have received some recognition in local history books and denominational and regional magazines.

In addition to the articles in the JNMA, five books have been written about specific African American hospitals in North Carolina. Two African American physicians who worked in North Carolina during the Jim Crow era wrote autobiographies. In his 1994 book, *Looking back: The way things were*, Dr. Milton Douglas Quigless described the founding and history of his Quigless Clinic in Tarboro. Dr. Hubert Eaton recorded his recollections and details of working at the Community Hospital in Wilmington in his book *Every man should try* (1984). Each of these autobiographies provide honest and detailed histories as well as commentary by physicians who were participants in providing health care and fighting racism in their communities, in North Carolina and in the nation. Two books have been written about Lincoln Hospital in Durham. In 2001, Dr. Preston Reynolds wrote *Durham's Lincoln Hospital*, and in 2013, Evelyn Wicker, RN, wrote *Voices: Lincoln Hospital School of Nursing*. Both are valuable sources about the history of the hospital. In 2008, local author O.W. Hawkins wrote *Pickford Sanitarium and R.C. Lawson Institute: Two former institutions of Southern Pines, North Carolina*, the only book about the Pickford Sanitarium in Southern Pines.

Several excellent books with broad histories of African American health and health care undergird this study. Byrd and Clayton's *An American health dilemma*, volumes 1 (2000) and 2 (2001) provide an almost encyclopedic basis for the study of African American health care from antiquity to the present day. In *Medical apartheid: The dark history of medical experimentation on Black Americans from Colonial times to the present* (2006), Dr. Harriet Washington chronicles the abuses faced by African Americans in medical research from the colonial era through the late 1900s. Dr. Edward Beardsley's (1987) *History of neglect: Health care for Blacks and mill workers in the twentieth-century south* analyzes the affects race and class had on the health of white mill workers and African Americans in Georgia, South Carolina and North Carolina. His research illustrates the failure of the southern medical, economic, and political establishment to respond to the suffering of the poor of all races. In her seminal work, *Black women in white*: *Racial conflict and cooperation in the nursing profession, 1890–1950*, Dr. Darlene Clark Hine examines the history of African Americans in the nursing profession. While her focus is on nurses and nursing, she also delves into the political, cultural, and economic milieu of African American hospitals and nurse-training institutions in the United States during the time period covered in this book. Very little of her work addresses North Carolina nurses of hospitals. Dr. Susan Smith's book *Sick and tired of being sick and tired: Black women's health activism in America, 1890–1950* highlights the roles of African American women activists in the public health movements in the first half of the 20th century. While centered on public health efforts, her analysis of local, state and federal health policy and their effects on African Americans contextualize the era of the rapid formation of African American hospitals in the United States.

Other authors have made significant contributions to understanding the health care issues facing African Americans in specific times and places. Four groundbreaking books on the health and health care of enslaved people, Fett's *Working cures: Healing, health, and power on southern slave plantations* (2002), Savitt's *Medicine and slavery: The diseases and health care of Blacks in Antebellum Virginia* (1981), Long's 2012, *Doctoring freedom: The politics of African American medical care in slavery and emancipation* and Covey's 2008 *African American Slave Medicine: Herbal and non-herbal treatments* provide comprehensive scholarship on this topic. Ward adds another dimension to the study of African American health care by documenting and discussing African American physicians who practiced in the era of legal racial segregation in his 2010 book *Black physicians in the Jim Crow south*. Beckford's 2011 *Biographical dictionary of American physicians of African ancestry, 1800–1920* also proved very useful for this study. Two books about specific aspects of hospital history inspired this book. The first, *Medicine in North Carolina: Essays in the history of medical science and medical service, 1524–1960* (1972) by Dorothy Long, was striking in its comprehensive scholarship yet limited descriptions of African American hospitals and sanatoria. Dr. Vanessa Gamble's *Making a place for ourselves: The Black hospital movement, 1920–1945* (1995), an important examination of African American hospitals in the United States early 20th century, touches on only a few of the largest African American hospitals in North Carolina. Dr. Karen Thomas's scholarly and valuable *Deluxe Jim Crow: Civil rights and American health policy, 1935–1954* (2011) highlights the health care situation for African Americans in North Carolina during a portion of the time period covered in this book.

There are two seminal books on the history of hospitals in the United States. One is Dr. Charles Rosenburg's exceptionally thoughtful *The care of strangers*. The other is Dr. Paul Starr's excellent *Social transformation of American medicine*. Neither fully discusses African American hospitals nor highlights the hospital history of North Carolina. Finally, Dr. C. Vann Woodward's 1974 influential work *The strange career of Jim Crow* provides an excellent explanation of the legal, social, economic and political forces that contributed to the enactment of laws in the southern states that forced the separation of the races, known as Jim Crow laws, in place from the end of Reconstruction until the Civil Rights movement of the 1950s and 1960s. While these and other scholars have written about African American physicians, nurses, patients and hospitals in the segregated south of the 1880s–1960s, no other work has focused solely on documenting the North Carolina African American hospitals during the Jim Crow era.

A Brief History of Hospitals in North Carolina Through 1900

Antebellum Era

In all times and in all cultures there exists a human inclination to care for others who are sick and injured. From the earliest days of North Carolina recorded history many have exemplified this impulse to care. Accounts from Native American sources, slave narratives and colonial records all describe relatives, servants and/or designated community healers tending to their ill and ailing family members and neighbors (Pollitt, 2014).

Like many other states, North Carolina had no general hospitals at the outbreak of the Civil War. The forerunner of the United States Public Health Service maintained Mt. Tirzah Hospital for Seaman near Wilmington, North Carolina, to quarantine sailors before they entered the city. The state founded the Dix Hill Asylum (later re-named Dix Hospital) in Raleigh in 1856 to treat white citizens with mental illness (Long, 1972; Pollitt, 2014). In the Antebellum Era, when white North Carolinians were ill or injured, they were usually cared for at home by mothers, wives, and sometimes slaves. A few plantation owners erected slave hospitals that offered rest and assorted tonics, poultices, and cures of the days (Fett, 2002). Cherokee and other Native Americans in North Carolina used plants and rituals passed down for untold generations to aid their ailing tribal members (Lefler, 2009).

The Civil War

At the outbreak of the Civil War, in the spring of 1861, no trained nurses or general hospitals and few physicians existed in the state of North Carolina. The leaders of the Confederacy were busy organizing a new government, establishing foreign relations and fighting the War. A common misconception was that the Civil War would be quickly and easily won. Because of this error in judgment, little provision was made for the care of wounded and sick soldiers. Instead, the Civil War produced an unprecedented number of sick and wounded soldiers creating a medical crisis.

The Confederate States of America quickly established 13 large military hospitals around North Carolina with the largest facilities in Charlotte, Fayetteville, Goldsboro, Raleigh, Salisbury, Wake Forest, Wilmington, and Wilson. Smaller, temporary hospitals—often run by local women and known as "wayside hospitals"—sprang up along railroad lines. Hotels, churches, and schools served as these makeshift hospitals. Some military camps established their own small hospitals for soldiers who fell ill during training. Despite the heroic efforts of doctors and nurses, conditions in Civil War hospitals were grim and overcrowded. Amputations were common and diseases spread rapidly. There were neither antibiotics to stop infections, nor immunization to prevent outbreaks of measles, tetanus, diphtheria, and other diseases that took more lives than the battlefields. None of these facilities allowed African American patients through their doors (Pollitt & Reese, 2002, Humphreys, 2013).

Early in the Civil War, much of coastal North Carolina fell to Union troops. Five Union hospitals were established in this area. These were the first hospitals in the state to offer more or less equal care to white and African American patients. In addition to Foster and Stanley hospitals in New Bern, Hammond Hospital in Beaufort, and the U.S. Army General Hospital for Colored Troops in Wilmington, smaller Union hospitals were located in Morehead City and on Hatteras Island (Giri, 2014; Hutchinson, 2002; Williams, 2011). Union troops captured Raleigh in the spring of 1865. Within days, the Union Provost Marshall ordered the first African American patient, a Union soldier, be admitted to Dix Hospital. Local African American residents soon followed. Dix Hospital was racially integrated until 1880 when the state built the North Carolina Asylum for Colored Insane (now Cherry Hospital) in Goldsboro, North Carolina (Dorothea Dix Hospital, 2014).

A great irony of the American Civil War is that its enormous toll on human health—over a million casualties, approximately 660,000 deaths from war and disease, 60,000 amputations, untold thousands suffering from a variety of physical and mental disorders—produced vast advances in scientific knowledge. Caring for hundreds of thousands of soldiers and civilians suffering from a wide array of ailments resulted in innovations in surgery, medicine, nursing, psychiatry, and public health. The benefits of hospitalization were evident during the Civil War. Many Civil War nurses incorporated ideas of sanitation, hygiene and nutrition advocated by British nurse Florence Nightingale in their nursing care, while many surgeons used new Listerian surgical techniques. Patients who received antiseptic surgeries had better outcomes than those receiving traditional surgery (Humphreys, 2013). Soldiers who convalesced in a clean environment with nutritious food and continuous oversight by skilled attendants fared much better than those in less healthy settings. These lessons would lead to the burgeoning of hospitals in North Carolina in the decades around the turn of the 20th century (Pollitt & Reese, 2002, Humphreys, 2013).

Freedmen's Bureau Hospitals

On March 3, 1865, close to the end of the Civil War, the federal government established the U.S. Bureau of Refugees, Freedmen and

Abandoned Lands. The Freedmen's Bureau, as the agency was popularly known, was created to help formerly enslaved people deal with the economic and social destruction and displacement caused by slavery and the Civil War. One function of the Freedmen's Bureau was the provision of health care services (Cimbala & Miller, 1999). In North Carolina, a medical division of the Freedmen's Bureau was created on June 16, 1865. It operated eight hospitals in the state—located in Wilmington, Raleigh, Beaufort, New Bern, Roanoke Island, Salisbury, Greensboro, and Morganton—usually in buildings that were former Confederate military hospitals. An additional Freedmen's Bureau clinic or dispensary was housed in the former Moravian, African American log church in Salem ("Negotiated segregation," n.d.). Their combined total capacity was 600 patients. Four full-time medical officers were assigned to the North Carolina Bureau's Medical Division, and another 14 contract surgeons were intermittently hired to treat and prevent the spread of communicable diseases (Pearson, 2002). Medical attendants were hired as needed with a peak of 45 employed in 1867. During the first full year of service, 24,130 people received hospital care, 11,525 were vaccinated against smallpox, and 598 women were given obstetrical care. In the 25 months of the North Carolina's Medical Division's existence, 40,343 people were treated and 4,798 of those died, resulting in a mortality rate of slightly over 10 percent (deRoulhac, 1909). In March 1868, the U.S. Congress voted to defund most of the functions of the Freedmen's Bureau, including its medical division. This left North Carolina with "no hospitals ... neither are there any medical men employed to attend to the poor, sick, and destitute freedmen" (Doherty [1868] as cited in Pearson, 2002).

From the closing of the Freedmen's Bureau hospitals in 1868 until the founding of St. Peter's Home and Hospital in Charlotte in 1876, no general hospitals existed in North Carolina. The North Carolina Board of Medicine's online timeline described the era:

> Patients and their families create their own remedies, or they seek medical assistance from herbalists, "granny women," or lay midwives. Medicine is practiced by anyone claiming to be a physician, and quackery is rampant. All doctors are generalists, and they usually travel to treat patients at patients' homes. A doctor may have a home office, which doubles as a compounding pharmacy. Technology is limited to what can be carried in a doctor's bag ["Doctors," n.d., p. 1].

These conditions were soon to change.

The Establishment of Early General Hospitals, 1876–1900

Hospitals, like all major social institutions, are complex organizations. They are both shaped by and help shape the political, economic and social milieus in which they are established. Most early hospitals were founded either by religious denominations and philanthropists fulfilling a benevolent impulse to care for others or by physicians seeking to provide optimal care for their patients while earning a living. For most of the 19th century, hospital patients were principally those who were socially isolated and/or unable to pay for private care (Mitchell, 1987). When middle- or upper-class persons fell ill, their families or servants usually nursed them at home. As Mitchell noted (1987), hospitals "were generally used by the poor and avoided by the middle class, who considered a bed among strangers as a last resort" (p. 162).

Before the acceptance of the germ theory of disease causation, and with few beneficial medications, laboratory tests, or body imaging equipment, hospitals in the 1880s and 1890s primarily provided a bedside attendant, a clean environment and regular meals. Rosenburg (1987) refers to this early stage of hospital development as the "domestic model." As advances in surgical techniques, the development of new medicines, and better understandings of the importance of hygiene and nutrition to health emerged in the early 1900s, hospitals began to evolve from charitable sanctuaries for the sick poor to modern scientific institutions. Patient outcomes for African American North Carolinians for both hospital births and for surgical procedures performed in operating rooms were far superior to those that occurred in patient's homes. This increased demand for hospital services, and in the decades around the turn of the 20th century, hospitals rapidly multiplied across the country.

The Founding of African American Hospitals

African American hospitals in North Carolina were established in similar patterns to hospitals across the country. Almost half, 39 of 85, of all hospitals founded in North Carolina between 1890 and 1910, and almost half of African American hospitals that existed during the

Jim Crow era, 18 out of 39, were privately owned by physicians (Hubbard, 2009). Noted nurse historian Dr. Eugene Tranbarger (2003) described the typical emergence of hospitals in North Carolina during this time:

> In the late 1800s, early 1900s, when two doctors opened a practice in the same town, the first thing they did was buy a hospital and open it and the second thing they did was start a school of nursing to provide the labor for the hospital [North Carolina Nursing History, 2003, n.p.].

The physician-owned African American health care facilities included Pickford Sanitarium in Southern Pines, Dr. Hargrave's Hospital in Wilson, Torrence Hospital, Circle Terrace Sanatorium and Blue Ridge hospitals in Asheville, Quality Hill Sanitarium in Monroe, Cordice Sanitarium and Trinity hospitals in Greensboro, Ray's Hospital and Williamson's Sanitarium in Winston-Salem, Dr. Erwin's Hospital in Gastonia, Rivera Clinic in Mount Olive, McCauley Private Hospital in Raleigh, Leary-Perry Hospital in Fayetteville, Susie Cheatham Memorial Hospital and Shaw Memorial Hospital in Oxford, Quigless Clinic in Tarboro, and Community Hospital in Wilmington.

Before Medicare, Medicaid, the Affordable Care Act or private insurance were available, the physicians who founded these hospitals had to buy equipment and supplies, pay nurses and other hospital employees and feed the patients before they made any income for themselves. Because most African Americans in North Carolina in the century after the Civil War were low-paid workers, they often contributed very little to offset their hospital bills. Therefore, most of these hospitals were small (had less than 50 beds), did not offer training programs for nurses or young physicians and were relatively short lived.

Until the enactment of the Civil Rights Act of 1964, medical education was not only segregated by race but also restricted almost totally to men, so very few women of any race became physicians or opened hospitals before the 1960s. The North Carolina census for 1880 lists 1,360 physicians and surgeons in the state and only 18 were women (Pollitt & Leonard, 1914). One exceptional white, female physician, Dr. Mary "Polly" Shuford, of Asheville founded the Shuford Clinic in the early 1940s to serve African Americans in and around Buncombe County, and played a major role in opening the Asheville Colored Hospital, 1943–1951. The only other example of white physicians owning and operating a hospital for African Americans was the Mercy Hospital in Wilson.

Following the biblical admonition to care for the poor and the sick, many churches and philanthropic individuals, acting benevolently within the norms of their day, opened hospitals with and for African American patients. Over a fourth or 10 of the 39 African American hospitals in North Carolina fall into this category. American Baptists launched the first African American hospital and only African American medical school in North Carolina on the campus of Shaw University in Raleigh in the 1880s. Episcopalians founded the Good Samaritan Hospital in Charlotte in 1891, St. Agnes Hospital in Raleigh in 1896 and Good Shepherd Hospital in New Bern in 1939. The Women's Missionary Union of the United Presbyterian Church owned and supported Jubilee Hospital in Henderson from 1911 to 1966.

Three major philanthropists donated large sums of money to create and sustain African American hospitals in North Carolina. Washington Duke, a tobacco magnate, and his heirs contributed tens of thousands of dollars for the founding and expansion of Lincoln Hospital in Durham. Winston-Salem industrialist R.J. Reynolds and his family gave liberally to both Slater Hospital, and later Kate B. Reynolds Memorial Hospital in Winston-Salem. Mrs. Mary Lynn Richardson, the widow of Lunsford

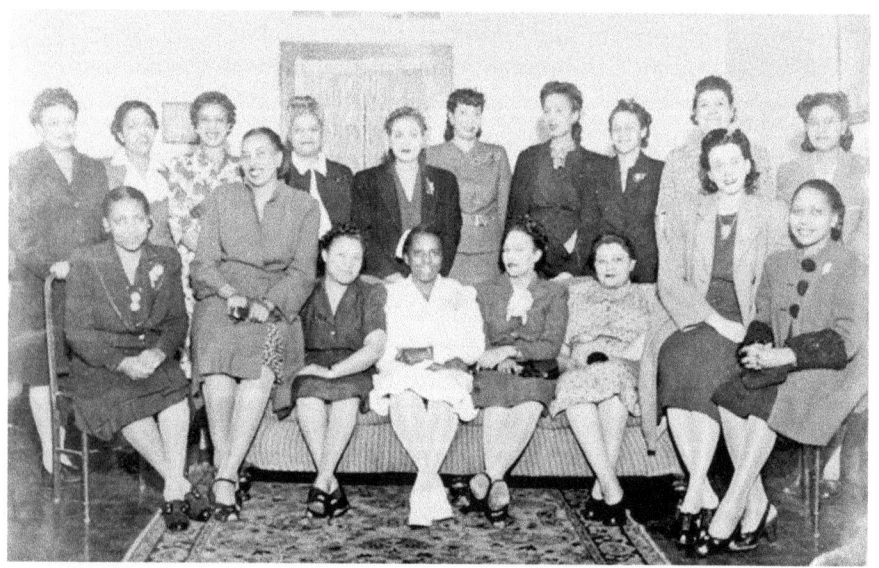

Ladies Auxiliary of the Good Samaritan Hospital, Charlotte, circa 1940s (courtesy Robinson-Spangler Carolina Room—Charlotte Mecklenburg Library).

Richardson, founder of the Vicks Chemical Company and inventor of Vicks Vapo-Rub, contributed $50,000 to a new African American hospital in Greensboro in 1927. After her donation, the hospital was named the L. Richardson Memorial Hospital, in his honor. Because these hospitals had significant financial backing from churches and/or philanthropists and strong ties to white religious and business leaders, they tended to be larger, better equipped, have more nursing schools and internship programs than those hospitals founded by African American physicians.

In addition to the physician-owned and benevolent hospitals, the state of North Carolina added three "Negro Divisions" to its already established public, tax-supported, white specialty hospitals. Cherry Hospital (originally named the Asylum for Colored Insane) opened in Goldsboro in 1880 to care for African Americans needing psychiatric treatment, the Negro Division of the State Tuberculosis Sanitarium was founded in 1922, and in 1925 the state established a Negro Division of the Orthopedic Hospital in Gaston County. The African American state-supported institutions opened later, had proportionally fewer beds and paid the African American professional staff less money than their white counterparts. However, they were supported by public funds and remained open as long as their white equivalents.

In addition to the 18 hospitals launched by African American physicians, the two founded by white physicians, the five founded by Protestant churches, the three supported by individual philanthropists and the three supported by the state of North Carolina, six additional African American hospitals served their communities during the Jim Crow era. Their founding stories are each unique and difficult to fit into any category.

In addition to the permanent hospitals discussed in this book, North Carolina was home to several "emergency hospitals" during both the influenza pandemic of 1918–1919, and during the extensive polio outbreaks in the 1940s. They were short lived and often funded and staffed by volunteers. Because of their transient nature, these hospitals are not included in this study.

Founding Dates of the First White and African American Hospitals in North Carolina's Largest Cities

Municipality	Name of Hospital	Primary Race Served	Year of Founding
Charlotte	Charlotte Home and Hospital	White	1876
Charlotte	Good Samaritan	African American	1891

Municipality	Name of Hospital	Primary Race Served	Year of Founding
Durham	Watts	White	1895
Durham	Lincoln	African American	1901
Asheville	Mission	White	1895
Asheville	Torrence	African American	1910
Winston (now Winston-Salem)	Grogan House/ Twin Cities	White	1887
Winston	Slater	African American	1901
Raleigh	Rex	White	1894
Raleigh	St. Agnes	African American	1896
Wilmington	James A. Walker	White	1901
Wilmington	Community	African American	1920
Greensboro	St. Leo's	White	1906
Greensboro	Cordice	African American	1914

The establishment of African American North Carolina hospitals fluctuated with social, political, legal and economic conditions through the decades of the 1880s through the 1950s. From 1880 to 1900, nine African American hospitals were established in North Carolina. Their founders reflect a cross section of the organizations and individuals who established hospitals. One was the state psychiatric Cherry Hospital, three were church related, two the result of individual philanthropy, one physician owned and one founded by a group of white and African American women in Charlotte working to improve their community.

As part of a nationwide boom in hospital construction, the majority of African American hospitals in North Carolina, 19 out of 39, opened in the twenty-year span from 1910 to 1930. The majority of these, 14 out of 19, were physician-owned institutions. One reason for this expansion is that Leonard Medical School (LMS), the first and only African American medical school in North Carolina, opened in 1882 and graduated its first class of six in 1886. As the number of LMS graduates grew, many stayed in North Carolina opening and staffing hospitals across the state. LMS closed in 1917, greatly diminishing the supply of African American physicians to open and staff African American hospitals.

Leonard Medical School Graduates Who Founded and/or Worked in African American Hospitals in North Carolina

Name of Graduate	Year of Graduation	Name of Hospital(s) Graduate Founded or Worked in
L.A. Scruggs	1886	Leonard Hospital—Raleigh, St. Agnes Hospital—Raleigh,

The Founding of African American Hospitals

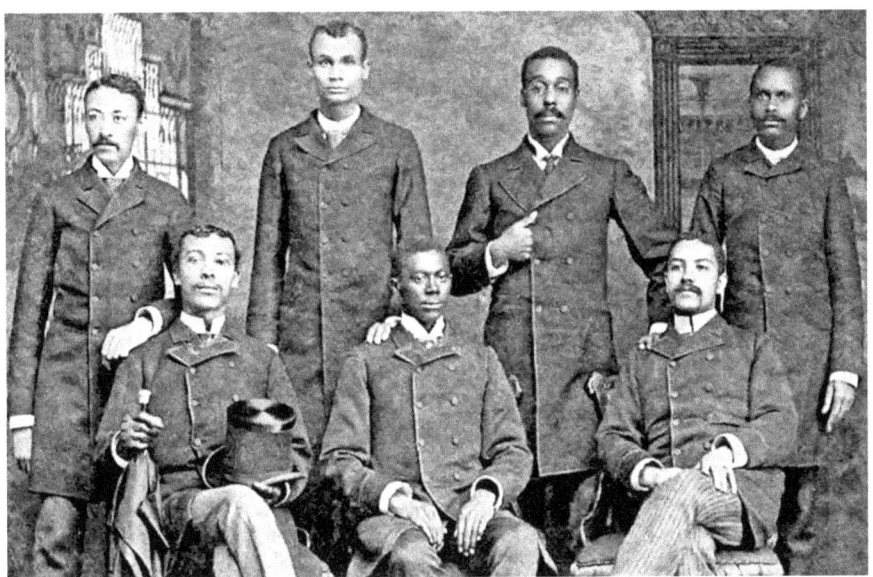

Graduating class, Leonard Medical School, Raleigh, 1889 (Wikimedia Commons).

Name of Graduate	Year of Graduation	Name of Hospital(s) Graduate Founded or Worked in
J.T. Williams	1886	Pickford Sanitarium—Southern Pines Union/Colored Hospital—Charlotte, NC, Good Samaritan Hospital—Charlotte
M.T. Pope	1886	Good Samaritan Hospital—Charlotte
H. Humphrey Hall	1887	Slater Hospital—Winston
Aaron McDuffie Moore	1888	Lincoln Hospital—Durham
Reuben Bryant	1889	Blue Ridge Hospital—Asheville
D.E. Caldwell	1890	Good Samaritan Hospital—Charlotte
John W. Jones	1891	Slater Hospital—Winston
Stanford Lee Warren	1895	Lincoln Hospital—Durham
John Sherman Massey	1896	Quality Hill Sanitarium—Monroe
Charles Shepard	1901	Lincoln Hospital—Durham
Frank S. Hargrave	1901	Slater Hospital—Winston, Dr. Hargrave's Hospital—Wilson
John Wakefield Walker	1902	Circle Terrace Sanitarium—

Name of Graduate	Year of Graduation	Name of Hospital(s) Graduate Founded or Worked in
John Earl Baxter	1905	Asheville, Negro Division–State Sanatorium—Sanatorium Jubilee Hospital
Joseph Napoleon Mills	1907	Lincoln Hospital—Durham
Nathaniel Edward Jackson	1907	Bigelow Hospital—Laurinburg
Alexander Hamilton Ray	1908	Ray's Hospital—Winston-Salem
Frank Avant	1908	Community Hospital—Wilmington
Herbert Jones Erwin	1908	Dr. Erwin's Hospital—Gastonia
Mathew Leary Perry	1908	Leary-Perry Hospital—Fayetteville
Chester Arthur Eaton	1910	Sanitarium—Fayetteville
William C. Strudwick	1910	Lincoln—Durham
Mathew D. Christmas	1911	Lincoln—Durham
Simon Powell	1912	Trinity Hospital—Greensboro
John Walcott Kay	1912	Community Hospital—Wilmington
John C. Williamson	1913	Williamson Sanitarium—Winston-Salem
Charles William Furlonge	1914	Furlonge Hospital—Smithfield
John Walker Holt	1917	Blue Ridge Hospital—Asheville

After the stock market crash of 1929, the economic hardships known as the Great Depression brought hospital construction to a virtual standstill. Neither African American physicians nor the state had enough money to undertake a hospital project. However, in the 1930s, three hospitals opened using private monies. Winston-Salem tobacco industrialist and philanthropist W.N. Reynolds made a considerable financial contribution so the Kate B. Reynolds Memorial Hospital could become a reality in 1938. One year later, the Episcopal Diocese of East Carolina opened a scaled-down version of their formerly imagined large and comprehensive Good Shepherd Hospital in New Bern in 1939. A group of white physicians in Wilson re-opened the formerly African American physician-owned Mercy Hospital.

Only four African American hospitals opened in North Carolina after the Great Depression. Three of these were physician owned and located in counties with few if any beds for African Americans. Despite these favorable conditions, before public funding for hospitalization, and when few African Americans had private insurance, one of these four hospitals, Leary-Perry Hospital in Fayetteville, closed the same summer it opened.

Military and Veteran's Administration (VA) Hospitals

Fayetteville is home to one of the largest Army bases in the United States, Fort Bragg. In 1941, at the start of World War II, and because of the wartime emergency, the Army opened its Nurse Corps to African American nurses. Army leaders viewed this as an experiment and limited the enrollment of African American nurses to 56. African American nurses were only allowed to care for African American service men. In April 1941, 24 African American nurses were assigned to Camp Livingston, Louisiana and another 24 to Fort Bragg. The Army had recently established segregated African American hospital wards on these two bases to treat ill and injured African American soldiers. Nurse Della Raney Jackson, a Lincoln Hospital School of Nursing graduate, was chosen to lead the Fort Bragg nurses (Black history month, 2009).

The Veteran's Administration's hospital system began after the Civil War when the federal government established National Homes for Disabled Volunteer Soldiers. These facilities were racially integrated from their founding in 1865 until the 1896 *Plessy v. Ferguson* Supreme Court decision allowed southern states to impose racial segregation in public accommodations. North Carolina was home to two VA hospitals before World War II. The first, Oteen (now Charles George), near Asheville, was founded shortly after World War I and implemented a "separate, but equal" policy for patient admissions, no African American professional staff were hired for over two decades. The VA hospital constructed in Fayetteville in 1939 followed the same policies as those found in the Asheville facility. VA hospitals built in Durham and Salisbury in the early 1950s also segregated patients by race and refused to employ African American physicians or nurses (Bielakowski, 2013).

The number of white and African American veterans with acute and chronic health conditions exploded after World War II. In 1930, there were 45 VA hospitals in the United States. By 1945, the number increased to 97 and in two years had grown again to 137 to meet the needs of returning World War II service men and women. It was extremely difficult to fully staff all of the new VA hospitals. At the same time, attitudes regarding racial segregation began changing after World War II. Many of these returning veterans along with others built the modern civil rights movement. The civil rights advocates and returning veterans found common cause in removing discriminatory policies in VA hospitals.

In 1948, President Harry Truman issued Executive Order 9981 outlawing racial discrimination in the federal workforce. This order included both military and VA hospitals across the country. Desegregation of the VA hospitals proceeded smoothly but took many years (Smith, 2005). In 1953, seven years after President Truman issued the Executive Order, Senator Adam Clayton Powell sent President Eisenhower a telegram noting that 27 VA hospitals still maintained racially segregated facilities. President Eisenhower took action and by 1954, all VA hospitals were fully integrated in patient room assignments and all had integrated professional staffs.

In the 1950s, many changes foreshadowed the racial integration of hospitals in North Carolina in the 1960s. Military and VA hospitals in Salisbury, Asheville, Fayetteville and Durham were the first hospitals in the state to employ physicians, nurses, laboratory technicians and others without regard to race. In the 1950s, many states, including nearby West Virginia and Kentucky, enacted state laws mandating tax-supported hospitals to care for anyone in need. During that same decade, the University of North Carolina School of Medicine began admitting African American students, and Dr. Hubert Eaton of Wilmington sued the white James Walker Hospital to become a member of the medical staff.

These events and others were the precursors to the successful elimination of legal segregation in hospital admissions and employment in the 1960s in North Carolina. While a small handful of the African American hospitals in North Carolina continued to provide care to African Americans and white patients after the mid–1960s, the era of African American hospitals was effectively over.

Nursing Education

Before 1950, all nursing education in North Carolina took place in hospital-based, diploma programs. All of the early nurse training programs in the state were primarily apprenticeships that catered to the demands of the hospital rather than the educational needs of students. Before 1920, students were often admitted at irregular intervals as vacancies occurred and needs arose for more help inside a hospital.

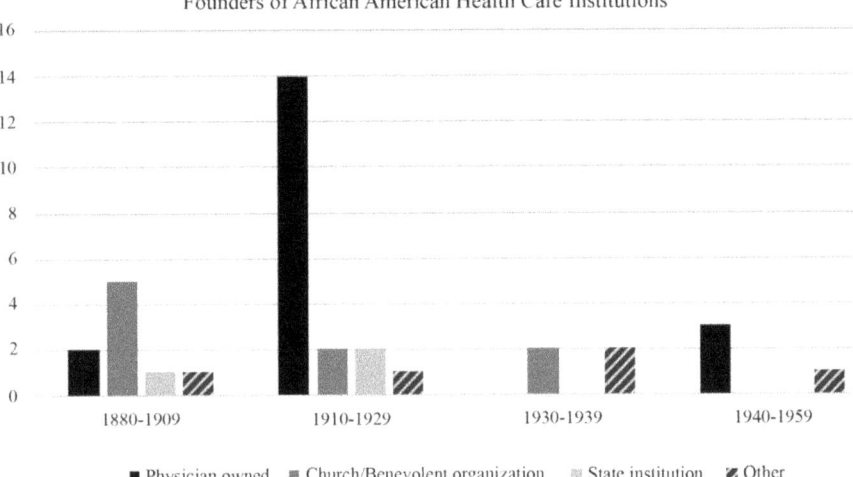

North Carolina hospitals typically ran on student labor, while graduate nurses worked in private duty (Pollitt, 2014).

Beginning in 1918, the North Carolina Board of Nursing (NCBON) established standards for nursing education programs, and only those students graduating from schools that earned an "A" or "B" rating from the NCBON could sit for the Registered Nurse examination. Students graduating from schools earning less than an "A" or "B" rating could be employed as "graduate nurses" or "trained nurses" but could not use the title Registered Nurse. Further, many occupational opportunities, such as working for the armed forces, the American Red Cross, and many public health agencies, were confined to those with the Registered Nurse credential. Registration became mandatory for nurses in North Carolina in 1965.

Almost a third or 11 out of the 39 African American hospitals in North Carolina had nursing education programs. The hospitals with accredited nursing programs were St. Agnes, Good Samaritan, Jubilee, Blue Ridge, Community, L. Richardson, Kate B. Reynolds, Lincoln, and the Negro Division of the State Sanitarium. Slater Hospital and McCauley Private Hospital ran smaller nursing education programs that were not accredited by the NCBON. Hundreds of graduates from these programs provided care inside African American hospitals, in Negro wards or wings of segregated white hospitals, in public health agencies and as educators of the next generation of nurses. Without

African American hospitals, there would have been no place for these nurses to learn their profession. The overall health of North Carolina's African American citizens would have declined from the already low levels they experienced.

Primarily for financial reasons, African American hospitals were built later, had fewer staff, were smaller, had less equipment and offered fewer services than white hospitals. However, many lives were saved, thousands of people's health improved, and hundreds of health care professionals were educated within their walls. Their contributions should not be forgotten.

Legal Segregation, Social Conditions and Medical Racism

From the colonization of the continent through the late 1960s, the primary determinant of the quantity and quality of health care people received was race. The 1896 U.S. Supreme Court Case *Plessy v. Ferguson* ushered in a period of legal racial segregation known as the Jim Crow era. Public, tax-supported entities, including public schools, parks, libraries, and hospitals, could be racially segregated as long as "separate but equal" facilities existed for each race. Private hospitals, tuberculosis sanitariums, and other health care facilities in North Carolina and across the country could legally ban African American patients from receiving any services. State-supported medical, dental, pharmacy, and nursing schools legally refused to admit African American students until U.S. Supreme Court cases forced their acceptance in the 1950s and 60s (Pollitt, 2016a, Pollitt, 2016b). Furthermore, health care institutions rarely hired African American physicians, nurses, or other health care professionals. In North Carolina, public hospitals, sanitaria, and clinics were strictly racially segregated but never equal in terms of supplies, equipment, personnel, or funding (Larkin, 1957).

In addition to limited access to health care, impoverished living conditions contributed to high rates of disease. A typical African American North Carolinian during this time period was described by Hemmingway (1980) as one who

> lived in a weather-beaten, unpainted, poorly ventilated shack, subsisted on a thoroughly inadequate diet and was disease ridden. Hook worms, pellagra and a

variety of exposure-induced ailments consistently plagued him, limiting his life expectancy rate [p. 213].

These conditions endured for decades. Dr. Thomas Parran (1938), the U.S. Surgeon General from 1936 to 1948, wrote that the African American's "house is the most miserable, his clothing the scantiest, and his food ration the most poorly balanced" of any group in the United States (p. 168). These racist laws and policies combined with sub-standard living conditions created a very unhealthy environment.

Racist scientific theories proclaimed African American's physiological and psychological inferiority. Many white physicians and scientists in the Jim Crow era believed that African Americans were Darwin's evolutionary "missing link" between apes and humans. Others erroneously claimed the African American race was weak, sickly, and biologically substandard when compared to all other races (Haller, 1971). In a 1903 article in the *Atlanta Journal-Record of Medicine*, Pittsburgh physician W.T. English described the bodies of African Americans as "a mass of minor defects and imperfections from the crown of the head to the soles of the feet" (p. 461).

Racist and unscientific medical writing lingered for decades. African Americans were often blamed for their condition. An article in the 1924–1926 biennial report of The North Carolina State Board of Charities and Public Welfare titled "The problem" states:

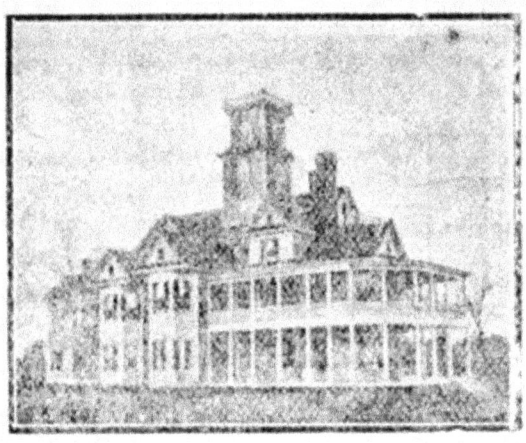

As the advertisement shows, African Americans were refused admission to many of the region's hospitals in the Jim Crow era (*Times Dispatch* [Richmond, Virginia], December 28, 1909).

> The masses of Negroes crowded in the mean quarters of North Carolina cities present problems in human depravity that can only be relieved by slow growth and the planting of desire among these people themselves to improve their condition.... Here are the hotbeds of disease, crime, and mental defectiveness that must be cleaned up if both races are not to suffer from the effect of those social ills in an ever increasingly degree.... It is inherently a question for the Negro to solve for himself.... There is a slothfulness, an ignorance, and a dreadful carelessness among them [p. 101].

Historian James Jones (1993) noted that many health care providers working for the U.S. Public Health Services in the infamous Tuskegee Study—the government-funded 40-year study of African American men with untreated syphilis—thought of their patents as a "notoriously syphilis soaked race" (p. 16). In addition to the assumption that African Americans were a physically inferior race, many white psychiatrists of the late 19th and early 20th centuries claimed emancipation from slavery caused mental illness in African Americans. An article by New Orleans physician Dr. Samuel Cartwright (1851) in *De Bow's Review of Southern and Western States* was illustrative of the times. He identified two psychiatric conditions found only in African Americans. The first was "Dysaethesai Aethiopica, or Hebetude of mind and obtuse sensibility of body—a disease peculiar to Negroes—called by overseers, 'Rascality'" (p. 1). Cartwright determined the cause of Dysaethesai Aethiopica/Rascality was emancipation from slavery, describing the condition as "the natural offspring of Negro liberty—the liberty to be idle, to wallow in filth, and to indulge in improper food and drinks" (p. 1). The second condition described by Dr. Cartwright was "Drapetomania, or the Disease causing Negroes to run away" (p. 1). In his article, Dr. Cartwright ascribed the desire for enslaved African Americans to escape their servitude to mental illness.

Racist legal, social, and scientific conditions created a horrifying zeitgeist for African Americans in North Carolina and throughout the United States. Living under these dire circumstances caused severe health problems, and without access to adequate and equitable health care, generations of African Americans unnecessarily suffered and died. Statistics reveal deep racial disparities in the health of North Carolinians in the 20th century but are inadequate to fully relate the grief and trauma experienced by many African Americans (Larkin, 1957).

20th-Century Statistics Documenting Health Disparities

Selected North Carolina health statistics from the early years of the 20th century paint a picture of the health inequities brought about by poor living conditions and discrimination in health care. The infant mortality rate per thousand births for white citizens in 1900 was 49.8 percent; for non-whites, it was 73.8 percent (Linder & Grove, 1947). In 1920, the death rate per thousand from the second leading cause of death, tuberculosis, was 92.1 percent for white North Carolinians and 171.1 percent for the states' African Americans (Steuart, 1922). That same year the overall life expectancy for white citizens was 56 years, which was a full decade longer than that of African Americans, who lived, on average, 46 years (Ewbank, 1987). An article in the March 1930 *North Carolina Health Bulletin* noted:

> The colored people in many of the cities and towns of North Carolina, as well as some in the country sections, have a death rate, especially among the infant population, sometimes approximating twice that of the white people in the same locality [North Carolina Board, 1930, p. 81].

Statistics from World War II disclose that 49 percent of white men were rejected from military service for health reasons, in comparison to the 71.5 percent of African American men who were found medically unfit to serve ("North Carolina Hospital," 1945). Although systematic collection of health data was not required until 1916—and even then, much was missed—these early statistics spotlight deep, racial disparities in every dimension of health measured. From infant mortality to average life span, the health disparities between white and African American citizens are startling.

Selected Causes of Death in North Carolina (5 Years and Older) in Which African Americans Died at Disproportionately High Rates, 1921

(Whites comprised approximately ⅔ of the state population while African Americans made up approximately ⅓ of the state population.)

Cause of Death	African American	White
Tuberculosis	1,208	1,425
Whooping Cough (Pertussis)	158	223

Cause of Death	African American	White
Pellagra	152	178
Typhoid Fever	151	155
Syphilis	80	22

Source: North Carolina Health Bulletin, June 1922, pp. 34–35.

Disparities in Hospital Beds by Race in the Mid–20th Century

One factor contributing to all health inequities that plagued North Carolina in the 20th century was racial discrimination in hospitalization. The quality and quantity of available hospital care impacts health throughout an individual's lifespan. Women and their infants who experienced physician-assisted hospital deliveries fared better in childbirth than those who delivered at home with poorly trained assistants. Surgical operations performed in antiseptic surroundings with adequate supplies, lighting, temperature, and personnel had better outcomes than those that lacked these basic commodities.

A state-wide survey published in 1944 reported that there were 48 hospitals in the state that banned African American patients, even in life-threatening emergencies. East of Rocky Mount, there were only 100 beds for the 300,000 African Americans who lived in the far eastern portion of the state. Fifty-five out of the 100 counties in North Carolina had no beds for African Americans at all ("North Carolina," 1945). In 1900, there was one white physician for every 300 white people, and one African American physician for every 9,000 African Americans in the state. Forty years later, the African American patient-to-physician ratio had slightly improved: there were 129 active African American physicians in North Carolina, resulting in a physician to patient ratio of 1 to 7,783 in 1940. Not a single hospital with segregated wards employed African American physicians ("North Carolina," 1945). During the time period covered in this book, African Americans in North Carolina never had equivalence on any measure of hospitalization with their fellow white citizens, resulting in an extreme disparity of healthcare access and quality of life.

**North Carolina Births by Race
and Type of Birth Attendant, 1937**

	White	African American
Number of births	53,748	24,564
% attended by a physician in a hospital	89.5%	35.3%
% attended by a lay midwife in the home	10.5%	64.7%

Source: North Carolina Health Bulletin, October 1939, p. 14.

The Duke Endowment

The Duke Endowment was the only southern philanthropy to make substantial contributions to African American hospitals in the first half of the 20th century. In 1924, Durham tobacco magnate and philanthropist James B. Duke established the Duke Endowment, a private foundation that funds health programs in North and South Carolina. From its founding in the 1920s through the 1950s, the Endowment's health spending had two primary purposes. The first was the establishment of hospitals in underserved areas and for underserved populations. The second was underwriting hospital costs for people in need, by donating one dollar per patient per day for charity care. Before the advent of publicly funded health programs, and before private health insurance was widespread, Endowment funds kept many hospitals open. The African American hospitals receiving Duke Endowment charity care payments in the 1920s and 1930s survived the Great Depression while several others, which were not recipients of these monies, closed during the hard economic times (Durden, 1998).

**Duke Endowment Financial Support to North Carolina
African American Hospitals, 1932, 1936 and 1944**

Name/Location of Hospital	1932	1936	1944
Community/Wilmington	$3,412	$5,772	$3,807
Gaston County Colored Hospital	$1,674		
Good Samaritan/Charlotte	$8,431	$10,183	$15,185
Good Shepherd/New Bern			$2,179
Jubilee/Henderson	$4,167	$4,104	$4,281
Lincoln/Durham	$20,130	$16,172	$10,743
Mercy/Wilson	$1,617		$3,846
L. Richardson/Greensboro	$5,049		$4,088
St. Agnes/Raleigh	$12,521	$15,554	$12,936
Susie Cheatham/Oxford	$1,540	$1,821	$1,199

The Duke Endowment collected and analyzed statistics relating to hospital care in the Carolinas from 1929 through the 1950s. The following table is taken from the Duke Endowment 1928 Annual Report. The chart illustrates the stark contrast of the distribution of hospital beds and physicians by race.

Negro Hospitalization

	Total	White Number	White Percent	Negro Number	Negro Percent
Population	2,938,000	2,062,476	70	875,524	30
Hospital Beds	7,626	6,405	84	1,221 (753 beds in segregated wards of white hospitals and 468 beds in African American hospitals)	16
Physicians	2,254	2,117	94	137	6
No. of Beds to 1,000 Persons	2.6		3		1.4
Population per Physician	1,304	974		6,391	

The Rosenwald Fund

In the early 1900s, Julius Rosenwald made a fortune as a part owner of the Sears, Roebuck Company, and in 1917 established the Rosenwald Fund (Fund) to distribute a portion of his wealth for "the well-being of mankind" (Embree & Waxman, 1949, p. 3). The first beneficiaries of his largess were schools for rural African American children in the southern states. Realizing the children's ability to succeed in school was being jeopardized by their many health issues, administrators of the Fund became interested in ameliorating the conditions that hampered the health of African Americans, including the lack of comprehensive, modern hospitals. Between 1928 and 1936, the Fund donated $562,000 to 16 African American hospitals including five in North Carolina. Good Samaritan Hospital in Charlotte and St. Agnes Hospital in Raleigh each received $15,000 while L. Richardson Memorial Hospital in Greensboro received $17,000 (Rice & Jones, 1994). Good Shepherd Hospital in New Bern was built using Fund monies along with significant donations from the Duke Endowment and various branches of the Episcopal Church. Finally, the Fund provided salaries for Lincoln Hospital in Durham to establish internship and residency programs in the mid–1930s.

One of the Fund's major goals was to encourage their beneficiaries to support African American personnel whenever possible as a means to promote professional integration in caring for patients and managing hospitals. However, neither the Duke Endowment nor the Rosenwald Fund required, nor expected, the African American and white hospitals they supported to be of equal caliber. Their financial assistance benefited many, while maintaining the racial status quo.

The North Carolina Medical Care Commission

Very few hospitals were constructed or expanded between 1929 and 1946 due to the Great Depression and the work force shortages caused by World War II. During World War II shocking statistics emerged in North Carolina. Soon after the war started, the State Board of Health had all boys in 11th and 12th grade examined for fitness for military duty. They found 85 percent had dental defects, 16 percent had vision problems, 16 percent were underweight, and 14 percent had enlarged tonsils. While 49 percent of the young white men who appeared before local draft boards were rejected as medically unfit for military service, 71 percent of African Americans were rejected for health reasons, the highest rejection rate in the country (Pollitt, 2014).

> In response to the public alarm over North Carolina's ranking forty-second in hospital beds per capita, forty-fifth in doctor-to-patient ratio, and highest in rates of World War II draft rejections, Governor J. Melvin Broughton, in 1943, proposed a comprehensive health plan for "more doctors, more hospitals, and more insurance [Kraus, 2006].

Responding to these startling health statistics, Governor Broughton assembled 50 health experts in a group he named the Medical Care

Commission. The Commission studied many aspects of health in the state. Some of their 1944 findings included that the death rate for African Americans was 146 percent that of the white death rate. There were no hospitals available to treat African Americans in 43 of the 100 counties. While there was one physician for every 1,938 white North Carolinians, there was only one doctor for every 6,916 African Americans (Silberman, 2010). One member, Dr. Selz Mayo, a rural sociologist, decried the effects the segregated hospital system had on health and on the North Carolina economy. He wrote:

> The people of North Carolina are too poor to afford bilateral health arrangements in health education, medical care facilities and in methods of paying for their services. At the same time, the state is too poor not to provide for one complete system of medical care. Two systems will mean lower standards and poorer services for both the white and Negro population [Mayo, 1945, p. 19].

All the data that had been collected by the Commission put the state in an advantageous position to receive federal dollars through the Hill-Burton Act a few years later (Silberman, 2010).

African American Hospital Beds in Segregated Hospitals by County, 1943

County	# of beds	County	# of beds
Alamance	60	Halifax	57
Anson	51	Harnett	46
Ashe	27	Haywood	4
Avery	2	Henderson	10
Beaufort	46	Iredell	12
Brunswick	21	Jackson	36
Burke	10	Johnston	62
Cabarrus	19	Lenoir	50
Caldwell	19	Lincoln	16
Carteret	25	McDowell	16
Catawba	43	Macon	9
Chatham	58	Mecklenburg	29
Cherokee	1	Moore	31
Columbus	55	Nash	18
Craven	15	New Hanover	4
Cumberland	31	Onslow	31
Davidson	43	Pasquotank	27
Durham	6	Pitt	60
Edgecombe	58	Polk	21
Forsythe	3	Randolph	36
Gaston	40	Richmond	56
Granville	51	Robeson	31
Guilford	21	Rockingham	46

County	# of beds	County	# of beds
Rowan	43	Union	51
Rutherford	36	Vance	25
Scotland	51	Wake	14
Stanley	24	Wayne	46
Surry	8	Wilkes	36
Transylvania	7	Wilson	31
Tyrell	29	Total	1,794

Source: North Carolina Medical Care Commission.

Number of Beds and Bassinets in African American Hospitals, December 1, 1947

Name of Hospital	Number of Bassinets	Number of Beds
Asheville Colored	6	20
Good Shepherd/New Bern	8	58
Lincoln/Durham	18	90
Gaston Colored	3	19
Susie Cheatham/Oxford	1	16
L. Richardson/Greensboro	8	58
Good Samaritan/Charlotte	21	100
Community/Wilmington	30	125
Jubilee/Henderson	5	39 (of which 10 were for tubercular patients)
McCauley Private/Raleigh	2	10
St. Agnes/Raleigh	18	90
Mercy/Wilson	2	61
Total	122	685

Source: North Carolina Medical Care Commission.

The Hospital Survey and Construction Act/ Hill-Burton Act

The health problems affecting North Carolina were echoed to some extent in almost every other state. Nationally, over six million men were rejected from serving in the armed forces due to mental and physical health problems. In response to health problems identified in draftees, soldiers, and veterans of World War II, in 1946 the U.S. Congress passed the Hospital Survey and Construction or Hill-Burton Act

(HBA). The "survey" portion of the Act provided three million dollars for states to assess the conditions and distribution of their current hospitals and for developing plans to address unmet hospital needs. Money was then allocated to the states to achieve a ratio of 4.5 general hospital beds per 1,000 people regardless of race. This did not mean integrating hospitals but only equalizing bed ratios for each state's population groups. States were allowed to use these monies to erect or improve segregated wings or wards of existing hospitals and/or to build new segregated hospital facilities (Thomas, 2011).

The Hill-Burton Act in North Carolina

North Carolina led the nation in the number of total projects, as well as segregated projects, completed under the Hill-Burton Act (HBA) (Rice & Jones, 1994). It was seventh in the number of new beds opened, and ninth in the amount of dollars spent (Wilkerson, 1992). Because the number of beds for African Americans in North Carolina was well below the HBA's target ratio, North Carolina received a disproportionate share of Hill-Burton funds and therefore the number of African American hospital beds dramatically increased (Thomas, 2006).

Of the 350 North Carolina projects funded by the HBA, 27 were for white-only facilities and four were for African American hospitals. Jubilee Hospital in Henderson was approved to use $196,000 in HBA funds along with local matching funds to construct a new 30-bed addition in 1957. L. Richardson Hospital in Greensboro received $77,000 in HBA funds which was matched with local funds to add an eight-bed unit. Durham's Lincoln Hospital used HBA monies to remodel portions of their facilities. Most HBA projects in North Carolina were used in white hospitals with segregated African American wards (Rice & Jones, 1994).

Lawsuits to End Hospital Segregation

As of 1961, no African American had ever been appointed to the North Carolina Mental Health Council, the State Board of Health, or the Medical, Dental or Nursing Boards of Examiners (Discrimination, 1963). While the North Carolina Nurse Association integrated its ranks in 1949, the North Carolina Medical Society did not fully integrate until 1965 (Halperin, 1988).

Early legal battles leading to the dismantling of segregation occurred in cases involving higher education, notably the 1938 *Missouri ex rel. Gaines v. Canada* case and later in cases involving public education including the groundbreaking 1954 *Brown v. Board of Education* decision. At the same time, African American physicians and dentists were using the court system to disassemble medical apartheid. Wilmington physician Hubert A. Eaton and Greensboro dentist George Simkins were courageous litigants and brave civil rights advocates.

Dr. Hubert Eaton was the first African American physician in North Carolina to sue a local hospital to try to end segregation. After Dr. Eaton finished his residency at Kate B. Reynolds Hospital in Winston-Salem, he moved to Wilmington, his wife's hometown. He joined the staff at Community Hospital, Wilmington's African American hospital (Mangus, 2015). Dr. Eaton soon discovered great disparities in facilities, equipment and staffing between Community Hospital and the local all-white James Walker Memorial Hospital (JWMH). In 1955, Dr. Eaton, Dr. Daniel Roane and Dr. Samuel Gray asked administrators at JWMH for the ability to care for their patients in the Negro wing of the hospital. Their request was denied. In 1956, the three physicians sued JWMH for violating their rights under the Fifth and Fourteenth Amendments to the U.S. Constitution. JWMH had never received Hill-Burton funds, but did receive a small amount of city and county funding and was tax-exempt. The physicians lost at every level because the courts did not consider JWMH a public institution and therefore were not subject to the same standards as tax-supported entities (Reynolds, 2004). While Dr. Eaton's lawsuit was making its way through the court system, a group of civil rights activists, led by dentist Dr. George Simkins, was suing segregated hospitals in Greensboro.

Simkins v. Moses H. Cone Memorial Hospital is a landmark decision by the 4th Circuit Court of Appeals and upheld by the U.S. Supreme Court that led to the legal elimination of segregated health care in North Carolina. Moses H. Cone Memorial Hospital (Cone) and Wesley Long Community Hospital (Long) in Greensboro had always practiced segregation. Neither hospital allowed African American physicians or dentists on their staffs. Both banned African Americans from their internship and residency training programs as well as their nursing schools. African American patients were admitted to Cone only under limited circumstances and were barred from Long altogether. However, the hospitals collectively received $2.8 million dollars in Hill-Burton funds for additions and improvements (Gamble, 1995).

In 1961, Dr. Simkins, who was also the president of the local chapter of the National Association for the Advancement of Colored People (NAACP), led a group of Greensboro African American physicians and dentists in petitioning both hospitals to end their discriminatory policies. Both refused. On February 12, 1962, Abraham Lincoln's birthday, Dr. Simkins and ten other Greensboro African American citizens, with attorney Conrad Pearson as their counsel, filed suit against Cone and Long hospitals. The American Public Health Association filed a brief on their behalf. The plaintiffs claimed that because the hospitals received almost three million dollars in Hill-Burton funds, they were at least semi-public institutions and therefore violated the plaintiffs' rights under the equal protection clauses of the Fifth and Fourteenth Amendments of the U.S. Constitution. Initially, the U.S. District Court found the hospitals were private, so they could continue their discriminatory policies (Gamble, 1995). Dr. Simkins and his allies appealed. In November 1963, the Fourth Circuit Court of Appeals held that racial segregation in hospitals using Hill-Burton Act monies for construction and expansion was unconstitutional. Hospitals using Hill-Burton funds in the region in which the Fourth Circuit Court had jurisdiction— Maryland, North Carolina, South Carolina, Virginia and West Virginia—could no longer legally use race as a criterion for admitting patients or hiring staff. Cone and Long hospitals appealed that decision to the U.S. Supreme Court which refused to hear arguments in the case and let the Fourth Circuit Court of Appeals ruling stand. The groundbreaking *Simkins v. Moses H. Cone Memorial Hospital* (*Simkins*) case was a major step in the elimination of segregation in North Carolina hospitals (Reynolds, 2004).

The Civil Rights Act of 1964

One of the most important pieces of federal legislation affecting segregation in North Carolina hospitals was Public Law 88–352 (78 Stat. 241) or the Civil Rights Act of 1964 (CRA). Title VI of the Civil Rights Act forbids discrimination on the basis of race, color, religion, sex, or national origin in all facilities including hospitals, nursing homes and other health care agencies receiving federal funds. It specifically reads:

> No person in the United States shall, on the ground of race, color, or national origin, be excluded from participation in, be denied the benefits of, or be subjected to discrimination under any program or activity receiving Federal financial assistance [Title VI of the Civil Rights Act of 1964, p. 1].

The CRA bans discriminatory admission and employment policies based on race in any hospital receiving any public money. The CRA reinforced the *Simkins* decision that African Americans had the legal right to be admitted to any hospital and work in any facility for which they were qualified. Like the *Brown v. Board of Education* Supreme Court decision that outlawed segregation in public schools, the *Simkins* case and the CRA of 1964 were implemented slowly and often met resistance across North Carolina (Reynolds, 2004).

Medicare and Medicaid

Unfortunately, these judicial and legislative victories did not quickly translate into non-racialized health care practices. Despite the *Simkins v. Moses H. Cone* court decision in 1963 and the Civil Rights Act of 1964, both which outlawed legally sanctioned racial segregation in hospitals and other health care agencies across the country, many North Carolina hospitals made no real strides toward integration. White hospital administrators knew that the *Brown v. Board of Education* decision of 1954, outlawing racial segregation in public schools, was rarely enforced a decade after its passage (Patterson & Freehling, 2001). Many white political and health care leaders in North Carolina saw no reason to quickly desegregate their facilities at the risk of alienating their client base. Although Title VI of the Civil Rights Act of 1964 prohibits organizations engaging in racial segregation from receiving federal funds, few hospitals in 1964 relied on federal monies for a significant amount of their budget. This was soon to change with the enactment of the Medicare and Medicaid additions to the Social Security Act on June 30, 1965 (Reynolds, 1997).

The Medicare program, enacted in 1965 and implemented in 1966, was a significant financial boon for hospitals across the country, providing health insurance for most United States citizens aged 65 and older. Medicaid was the largest source of funding for medical and health-related services for America's poorest people. Together these programs would grow to account for a substantial portion of hospital revenue by the late 1960s (Friedman, 1990). Dr. David Smith (2005), a Temple University professor of health care management, noted:

> Medicare payments were large, essential, and generous. Hospitals were reimbursed on a cost-plus basis. Combined with Medicaid dollars, the federal dollars would account for the majority of hospitals' income. Ultimately, hospitals had to choose between affluence through compliance [with racial desegregation laws] or bankruptcy [p. 13].

In 1966, the U.S. Department of Health, Education and Welfare created the Office for Equal Health Opportunity (OEHO) to track hospital compliance with the new civil rights legislation. Three hundred OEHO inspectors made visits to southern hospitals, and when they found signs of segregation in patient care areas or employment, Medicare and Medicaid funding to the offending hospital could be, and sometimes was, terminated. For instance, Rex Hospital, the oldest white hospital in Raleigh, was investigated and found to be out of compliance with the Civil Rights Act in 1966. The hospital lost Medicare funding for a year, but since it was in compliance during an investigatory visit in 1967, funding was restored (Halperin, 1988). Almost all hospital administrators chose government funds over segregation. More than 1,000 segregated hospitals, including almost all hospitals in North Carolina, quietly and uneventfully integrated their staffs, cafeterias, waiting rooms, and hospital floors in less than four months in the spring and summer of 1966 (Beardsley, 1986).

The importance of hospital care is perhaps illustrated most dramatically in maternal and infant death statistics for non-whites in North Carolina in 1963, when segregation was required, compared to the same statistics in 1969, several years after hospitals were integrated and funding for care for low income women was more available. Infant (children from birth to 1 year of age) deaths decreased from an alarming 50.8 percent to 37.1 percent for non-whites. Maternal death rates for non-whites were cut in half, from 13.1 deaths per 1,000 births in 1963 to 6.6 deaths per 1,000 women in 1969. Many other health outcomes improved for non-whites as hospital care became more available and affordable (Halperin, 1988).

Conclusion

The system of medical apartheid, implemented in North Carolina in 1880, remained in place until the Civil Rights movement of the 1960s. While some white hospitals had a limited number of "Colored" beds, they were usually in dark, damp basements or poorly heated attics where patients were attended by unfamiliar white physicians and nurses with varying degrees of respect. Reflecting on common practices in a 1999 oral history interview, African American nurse's aide Mrs. Mabel Williams recalled conditions at the Ellen Fitzgerald Hospital in Monroe during segregation. African American patients were treated in the basement, and newborn infants spent their first hours in the basement's utility room, the same room where nurses emptied bedpans. Neglect was not limited to African American infants; Williams recalls that standards were very lax in the African American section of the hospital, with nurses performing many duties restricted to doctors in the white section on the upper floors (Oral history, 1999). Usually white hospitals that maintained facilities for African Americans had one ward for males and one for females, so a woman who had recently given birth might be placed next to a tubercular patient or someone recovering from surgery. Little thought was given to infection control or hygiene (Cobb, 1947).

Under these dire circumstances, brave African American physicians, often with help from white allies, erected their own hospitals to provide care with dignity and respect for anyone in need. African American hospitals not only treated people in their communities and educated young people into health professions, but also served as beacons of racial pride and mechanisms for social uplift. These health care leaders heeded the words of Dr. Daniel Hale Williams, the founder of Provident Hospital and Nurse Training School in Chicago, who exhorted his colleagues at a meeting in Nashville in 1900:

> In view of this cruel ostracism, affecting so vitally the race, our duty seems plain, institute Hospitals and [medical and nursing] Training Schools. Let us no longer sit idly and inanely deploring existing conditions. Let us not waste time trying to effect changes or modifications in the institutions unfriendly to us, but rather let us seek to promote the doctrine of helping and stimulating our race [as cited in Gamble, 1995, p. 3].

In the spirit of Dr. William's poignant declaration, North Carolina African American physicians and nurses, sometimes with white allies, established at least 39 hospitals and other health care facilities during the period of racially sanctioned segregation. This book highlights the work of these courageous pioneers of equitable healthcare in the state. In North Carolina, the most important institution contributing to improved African American health care in the 20th century was Leonard Medical School on the campus of Shaw University in Raleigh.

PART II

The Health Care Facilities

Raleigh, Wake County

Wake County, in the central piedmont section of the state, was originally home to the Sissipahaw and Occaneechi tribes. In the early 1700s, Scots-Irish and British pioneers, with enslaved Africans, drove out the Native Americans and began farming the land (Powell, 2006). In 1860, a year before the Civil War started, there were 28,627 residents in Wake County. Of those, 16,470 or 62 percent were white, 10,738 enslaved and 1,494 were free African Americans (Ptak, 2010).

In 1900, Raleigh, North Carolina, was a medium-sized Southern town and the capital city. With a population of 13,643, Raleigh was the state's fifth largest city. Approximately a third of the population was African American. It was a commercial, educational, and governmental center. Raleigh was home to six colleges and junior colleges: five were private, and one was a large state university. There were three private white women's colleges, one large state supported school for white men, and two African American colleges, the Baptist Shaw University and St. Augustine's University sponsored by the Episcopal Church (Murray, 1983).

In the early 20th century, Raleigh was home to over 50 African American small businesses, including a newspaper, restaurants, funeral homes, and barber shops. There were a wide variety of African American churches and civic organizations. The Raleigh African American community ranged from manual laborers living and working in substandard, even hazardous environments, to professionals living in large, modern homes (Mattson, 1988).

Raleigh's Shaw University was home to Leonard Hospital, the first African American hospital in North Carolina; this facility also served as the clinical training site for Leonard Medical School's students, the only African American medical school in North Carolina. Additionally, Raleigh was home to the state's first African American school of nursing at St. Agnes Hospital on the campus of St. Augustine University. To treat African Americans who could afford a more personal relationship with their physician and private rooms, Dr. Lewyn McCauley, a graduate of Leonard Medical School and professor at the St. Agnes School of Nursing, opened a small, private hospital. Following are brief sketches of each of these pioneering institutions.

Leonard Hospital and Medical School, 1885–1918

On December 1, 1865, less than 8 months after the Civil War ended, Union Army veteran, Baptist preacher, and Massachusetts native the Rev. Henry Martin Tupper and his wife Sarah Leonard Tupper moved to Raleigh, North Carolina, to establish the school that became Shaw University (Morehouse, 1890). They were supported by the American Baptist Home Mission Society, whose goal was "to preach the Gospel, establish churches and give support and ministry to the unchurched and destitute" (Whitted, 1908, p. 5). The school quickly became a success with an increasing enrollment and a growing campus. Academics initially focused on the fundamentals of literacy and numeracy with advanced courses aimed at educating future Baptist preachers ("Shaw Celebrates," 2014).

The Reverend Tupper, as well as other Shaw supporters, was responsive to the needs of the times. In 1876, he noted, "The colored people at present are without educated Physicians, and are thus subject to all manner of quackery and imposition, and many suffer and die for want of attention" (as cited in Zogry, 2008, p. 145). Reacting to these dismal conditions, Sarah Tupper's brother, Judson Wade Leonard, donated money to create the first medical school for African Americans in North Carolina at Shaw University. It was also the first four-year medical school in the United States (Carter, 1973). Leonard Medical School (LMS) remained the only North Carolina medical school that accepted African American students until 1951 when the University of North Carolina at Chapel Hill School of Medicine accepted Edward O. Diggs of Winston-Salem ("3 race students," 1951).

The Leonard Medical Center's first building Leonard Hall, named

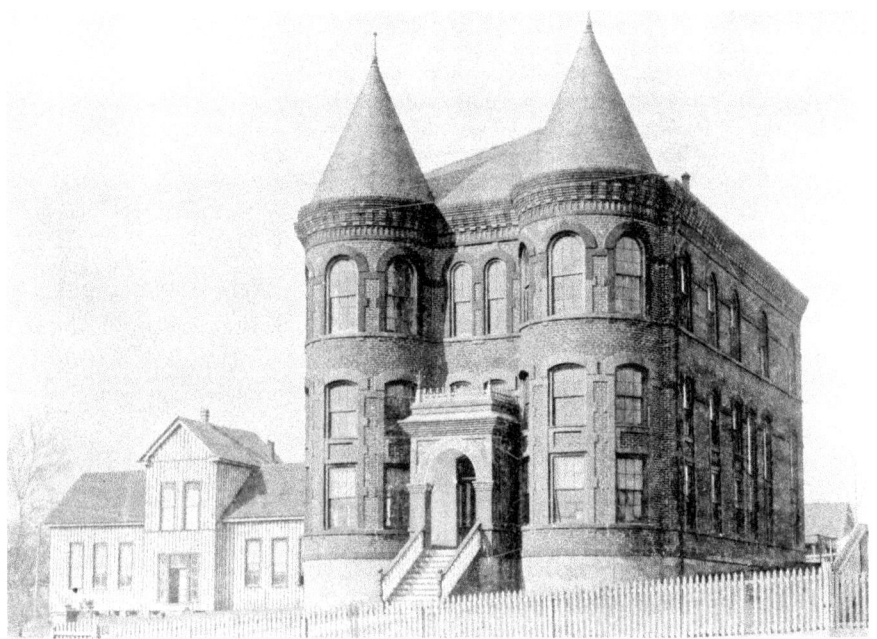

Leonard Medical School in Raleigh, operated from 1882 to 1914 (Library of Congress).

in recognition of Leonard's generous support, opened in 1882 and housed classrooms, laboratories, and offices (Blackburn, 2006). Initially, in the 1880s and 1890s the school and hospital were in session for about five months a year from October through early April, giving students time to earn money to pay for their education. In 1906 the Board of Trustees lengthened the academic year for the pharmacy and medical schools to eight months. The Leonard Medical School catalog for the 1907–1908 academic year illustrates the academic rigor necessary to be admitted to, and to graduate from LMS.

> Preliminary Course.
> If a student fails to pass a satisfactory entrance examination, he will be expected to spend a sufficient time in the preliminary studies to qualify himself for the regular course. This will include instruction in Latin, Botany, Physics, Zoology, Chemistry, Physiology, and the use of the microscope. These branches will enable the student to pursue with greater facility the Medical Science.
> Examinations and Graduations.
> The following will be the order of the examination in the Graded Course: At the end of the first year, Materia Medica [pharmacology], General Chemistry,

Anatomy and Physiology; at the end of the second, Anatomy, Physiology and Medical Chemistry; at the end of the third, Therapeutics, Obstetrics, the Principles and Practice of Medicine and Surgery; at the end of the fourth year, a final examination of all the branches pursued during the course, occupying the last week of the term. The examinations will be written as well as oral, and will be marked on the scale of one hundred. A failure to receive 80 per cent in any branch will require that study to be repeated the next year, and the student to be re-examined in the same at the close of the year [Leonard Medical School catalog, 1907, p. 21].

Leonard's first class of six men—M.S.G. Abbot, James Bugg, M.T. Pope, A.T. Prince, L.A. Scruggs, and J.T. Williams—began their studies in October 1882, and all passed the North Carolina Board of Medicine examination in 1886 and began their medical practices (Savitt, 1999).

Medical education at Shaw took a major leap forward when Leonard Medical School Hospital (LMSH) opened on January 10, 1885 (Savitt, 1984). Not only did students now have a hospital in which to practice their clinical skills, but the African American people of Raleigh and surrounding Wake County also had a hospital staffed largely by African American medical students and nurses. The hospital had 25 beds in three patient wards (Savitt, 1984).

Several brief, optimistic items appeared in local newspapers in the 1880s and 1890s. Typical of these articles are the two excerpted below. The following piece, published on October 1, 1886, was published shortly after the hospital was completed: "Leonard Medical School opens November 1st with every prospect of a prosperous year.... The school is in a condition to give completeness and unity to the course of study not hitherto attained" ("Leonard Medical School," 1886, p. 2). Another article, entitled "The closing session of Leonard Medical School," celebrated the accomplishments of the second graduating class and was published on April 13, 1887, in *Biblical Recorder*:

> The Medical Department reaches a high standard every session, and from the increased facilities and large attendance of pupils from last session, it would seem that the medical profession is soon to wield a great power in elevating suffering humanity among the colored people of this country and perhaps the mother country, Africa [p. 2].

Way and McBrayer noted the aspirations of the founders of LMS in their 1928 book *Medical colleges in North Carolina*:

> A worthy ambition characterized the beginning of the school: "In making our second announcement we will state that it is our aim to follow as closely as

possible the curriculum of study as pursued at Harvard and other first-class medical schools [p. 142].

Community awareness and support of the hospital was spread through articles such as these and other publications; this support was vital to the hospitals' growth and achievements.

In addition to newspaper articles, statistics reveal how beneficial LMSH was to the local community. The *Report to the Raleigh Mayor and Board of Alderman*, dated March 18, 1890, informed its readers that LMSH was open from November 1, 1889, through April 1, 1890, the same time the medical school was in session. During those five months, 39 patients were treated. Of the 20 acute cases admitted, 18 were cured. There were 18 patients admitted with chronic diseases of which six were cured and five improved. All seven surgeries performed were successful. Seven women gave birth, and all the mothers and babies survived. In addition, over 100 people received various services as outpatients (Scruggs, 1890). Without LMSH and its newly trained African American physicians, many of these patients would not have received quality care, increasing their risk of fatality from illness, surgery or child birth. The chart below details where LMS graduates practiced in 1895 and 1905. Most of the areas in which they set up medical practices had few, if any, African American physicians before they arrived. The impact of LMS was felt across the United States and in foreign countries.

Leonard Hospital Graduates' Locations of Practice After Graduation, 1895 and 1905

State	1895	1905
Alabama	1	10
Arkansas	2	4
California		1
Colorado		1
District of Columbia		2
Georgia	7	16
Florida	2	2
Illinois		1
Maryland		3
Massachusetts		5
Mississippi		1
New Jersey		5
New Mexico		1
New York		2
North Carolina	19	45

State	1895	1905
Ohio		1
Pennsylvania		6
Rhode Island		1
South Carolina	9	17
Virginia	9	48
West Virginia	2	8
British West Indies		2
South Africa		1
Known to be deceased		15
Total	51	198

LMS administrators and faculty strove to maintain high standards for medical education. The 1907–1908 LMS catalog announced:

> In the Department of Anatomy and Physiology many additions have been made. The school has now almost the complete set of Auzoux and Bock Steger anatomical models, which have been imported from Paris especially for our use.
>
> Accessories for the microscope have been obtained, so that the study of Histology and Microscopical Pathology can be pursued.
>
> Models for the study of Obstetrics have been secured, and further additions in the way of models and instruments will be made from time to time [Leonard Medical School catalog, 1907, p. 24].

Leonard Hospital frequently faced financial problems and was only opened during the months the medical school was in session. Despite these obstacles, it rendered valuable services to its constituencies. For its 34 years (1885–1919) of existence, LMSH was a cherished institution for many in Raleigh and surrounding Wake County (Savitt, 1984). The facility continued to valiantly serve the needs of African Americans seeking a medical education, as well as the African American people of central North Carolina who sought hospitalization for surgery, childbirth, and medical care. As the 20th century dawned, a new era in medical education emerged.

As medical education developed in the 20th century, after graduating from medical school, physicians planning to specialize in a specific area, such as surgery, obstetrics or pediatrics, undertook a hospital-based internship. After the internship, some furthered their training through a residency program. Not all hospitals had internship and residency programs, and those that did usually had fewer spots than there were graduates seeking the positions. In order for a hospital to offer these programs, there had to be enough staff to train the interns and residents as well as facilities and equipment to teach state-of-the-art care (Rice & Jones, 1994).

Until the enactment of civil rights laws, no all-white and few integrated hospitals in the country, and none in North Carolina, accepted African American doctors into their internships and residency programs. In 1930 there was not a single African American resident in the United States (Ward, 2003). In 1931, there were 93 African American interns in the country; eight of them were in North Carolina—three at Lincoln Hospital in Durham, three at St. Agnes Hospital in Raleigh and two at L. Richardson Memorial Hospital in Greensboro. While the number of African American interns increased to 120 by 1936 nation-wide, the number in North Carolina remained at eight (Rice & Jones, 1994). Community Hospital in Wilmington and Kate B. Reynolds Memorial Hospital in Winston-Salem began internship programs after World War II while Lincoln Hospital in Durham and St. Agnes Hospital in Raleigh began residency programs. (Thomas, 2011). These limited opportunities for medical school graduates meant few African American physicians received training to become specialists. This situation was yet another reason many African American patients in North Carolina received care inferior to white patients who could be cared for by white physicians with many years of specialized training.

FLEXNER REPORT OF 1910

A watershed event in medical education occurred in 1910 with the publication of the *Medical education in the United States and Canada: A report to the Carnegie foundation for the advancement of teaching* (Flexner, 1910), commonly known as the Flexner Report. This report was a catalyst for the demise of Leonard Medical School, less than a decade after the report's publication.

Without nationally accepted standards, the quality of medical schools varied wildly in the decades around the turn of the 20th century. The recently formed American Medical Association, the segregated, white-only, physicians' professional association, created the Council on Medical Education in 1904 to deal with the "enormous overproduction of uneducated and ill trained medical practitioners" (Pritchett, 1910, p. 7). Criteria for admission and graduation, quality of faculty, holdings in libraries, equipment in laboratories, and use of clinical sites ranged from abominable to excellent (Beck, 2004). In 1907, funding was secured from the Carnegie Foundation for the Advancement of Teaching to undertake a national survey of medical schools with an eye towards setting minimum standards and making recommendations for improvements. Abraham Flexner, an educator from Kentucky, was hired to undertake the work. His report, issued in 1910, recommended about half of the medical schools in the country be closed. In the special section about the seven African American schools then operating, he wrote: "The Negro needs good schools, not many schools ... five are at this moment in no position to make any contribution of value" to medical education (p. 180). He recommended only Meharry Medical School in Nashville and Freedmen's Hospital Medical School in Washington, D.C., remain open. Flexner believed that African Americans were unable to fully function as physicians and needed the supervision of White colleagues. He noted, "The Negro must be educated not only for his sake, but for ours.... Ten million of them live in close contact with 60 million whites" (Flexner, 1910 p. 180). By 1920, largely as the result of the Flexner report, the number of medical schools in the United States had been reduced from 155 to 85. Only two out of the seven existing African American medical schools survived (Beck, 2004).

Flexner visited LMSH in February of 1909. His entire report on and comments about LMSH appeared as follows:

RALEIGH: Population 20,533
LEONARD MEDICAL SCHOOL, Colored, Organized 1882.
Entrance requirement: Less than four-year high school education.
Attendance: 125
Teaching staff: 9, of whom 8 are professors, one of other grade.
Resources available for maintenance: Mainly fees and contributions, amounting to $4721, practically all of which is paid to practitioner teachers. There are no library, no museum, and no teaching accessories. It is evident that the policy of paying practitioners has absorbed the resources of a school that exists for purely philanthropic objects.
Clinical facilities: These are hardly more than nominal. The school has access to a sixteen-bed hospital, containing at the time of the visit three patients. There is no dispensary at all. About thirty thousand dollars are, however, now available for building hospital and improving laboratories.
A word as to the colored school at Raleigh: This is a philanthropic enterprise that has been operating for well-nigh thirty years and has nothing in the way of plant to show for it. Its income ought to have been spent within; it has gone outside, to reimburse practitioners who supposed themselves assisting in a philanthropic work. Real philanthropy would have taken a very different course. As a matter of fact, Raleigh cannot, except at great expense, maintain clinical teaching. The way to help the negro is to help the two medical schools that have a chance to become efficient, Howard at Washington, Meharry at Nashville.
Date of visit: February 1909 [Flexner, 1910, pp. 281–282].

Consequences of the Flexner Report

The consequences of Flexner's lack of support for Leonard Hospital ultimately led to the facility's closing. The implementation of the Flexner Report, just 48 years after the Emancipation Proclamation, obstructed opportunities for African Americans pursuing medical education and restricted the production of physicians capable of addressing the health needs of over 10 percent of the nation's and 33 percent of North Carolina's population.

In an effort to remain open and meet the new higher standards expounded in the Flexner Report, the American Baptist Home Missionary Society provided $30,000 for a new hospital building and other improvements (Johnson & Murray, 2008). Leonard Hospital opened its new building on February 5, 1912 (Emerson, 1913). Emerson (1913) described the new 80-bed hospital as "modern in every respect, having been constructed in accordance with the latest approved methods of heating, lighting and sanitation" (p. 87). In addition to a men's and women's ward, the new hospital had a reception area, a superintendent's office, an anesthetizing room, a surgical supply room, an operating room, a recovery room, several private rooms, a maternity ward, and a children's ward "furnished by Mrs. Josephus Daniels, wife of the Secretary of the Navy" (Emerson, 1913, p. 87). Hospital staff included a hospital superintendent, a house physician, a head nurse, four staff nurses, one or more interns, an orderly, and a housekeeper. The nurses cooked and served the patients food. Fees were $5 for care in a ward bed and $10 a week for a private room. In the first year, 300 patients were admitted and 44 operations were performed (Emerson, 1913). Leaders of Shaw University struggled to find the funds to upgrade and maintain the medical school sufficiently to earn an "A" rating from the American Medical Association. Terms were lengthened from five to eight months, admission standards were raised, additional supplies including a microscope were purchased for the laboratory, and more faculty and courses were added. Each of these improvements increased the budget. The Raleigh Academy of Medicine, the association of the white physicians in Raleigh, passed a resolution in support of LMS. The *Raleigh News and Observer* printed their endorsement of LMS in its November 8, 1917, edition:

> That we endorse the Leonard Medical School of Shaw University in the city of Raleigh, in its efforts to raise its standards. That we commend the school to the

Council on Medical Education of the American Medical Association, as worthy of admission to the list of Class "A" colleges. That we join with this school, the Meharry Medical College and the Medical Department of Howard University in asking the cooperation of the Southern Medical Association for the purpose of promoting Negro medical education in the south and in an appeal to the General Education Board and the American Baptist Home Mission Society, for the continuation of their support for the work ["Raleigh Doctors," 1917, p. 2].

Unfortunately, the Rockefeller General Education Board and other philanthropists gave their support to both Meharry Medical College and the Medical Department at Howard University, leaving LMS without a major benefactor. In 1914, LMS reduced its program to a basic two-year science curriculum to prepare students to attend other medical schools, and in 1918, closed its doors (Savitt, 1999).

Although LMS was unable to meet all of the standards required by the Flexner Report, its demise led to poorer health outcomes for African American people in North Carolina and the south. Without a steady supply of African American physicians to treat patients, and to open African American hospitals and nursing schools, access to quality health care became more difficult in the mid–20th century than it was in 1900. By 1920, only two medical schools, Meharry Medical College in Nashville and Howard University in Washington, D.C., graduated over 90 percent of the country's African American physicians. Almost 40 percent of those African American physicians practiced in seven Northern states with less than 20 percent of the country's African American population, leaving broad areas of the American south without any African American physicians to provide care. None of the 26 state-supported medical schools in the old Confederacy admitted African American students until the 1960s. A handful of medical schools in the rest of the country admitted a limited number of African American students, but costs, travel and lack of sound educational preparation in segregated public schools were deterrents for many aspiring African American physicians (Ward, 2003).

The 480 LMS graduates worked across North Carolina, the country, and even in parts of Africa providing care, erecting hospitals, and starting nursing schools (Savitt, 1984). These contributions to the health of African Americans in North Carolina during the Jim Crow era are incalculable, especially considering that most white health care professionals practiced racial exclusion, discrimination, and neglect. While the Baptist Leonard Medical School was a pioneer in educating African American physicians, only a mile or two away, St. Augustine

College was establishing the first nursing school for African American women in North Carolina at its St. Agnes Hospital.

St. Agnes Hospital and School of Nursing, 1896–1960

After the Civil War, most protestant denominations sponsored home missionaries to "uplift" the newly emancipated freedmen and women through religion and education. While the American Baptists were supporting Shaw University and Leonard Medical School, the Episcopalians founded St. Augustine School (now University) in Raleigh. In 1867, the Rev. Aaron Burris Hunter and his wife Sarah—both white, northern, home missionaries—arrived in Raleigh, North Carolina, to teach at St. Augustine's School. Students from the capital city of Raleigh and surrounding counties came to St. Augustine's to get an elementary and high school education and to study for the Episcopal ministry. The school was very successful and grew through the decades in both number of students enrolled and variety of programs offered (Roundtree, 2002). The Hunters, like the Tuppers at Shaw University, recognized the impact poor health, partially due to the lack of African American physicians, nurses, and hospitals, had on the lives of local African American citizens (Delany, 1930). Neither the "Colored Annex" at the local Rex Hospital nor Leonard Hospital, which was only open from November through March, completely met the health care needs of the African American community in and around Wake County (Williams, 1994). The Hunters and others wanted to establish a year-round African American hospital where patients could receive a full range of services in a respectful environment.

Pursuing this dream, in 1885, Sara Hunter addressed the Women's Auxiliary of the Protestant Episcopal Church at its national meeting. She stressed the need to add a hospital and nursing school to the campus at St. Augustine, then asking for donations. Mr. T. L. Collins of California heard about Hunter's appeal and donated $600 in memory of his recently departed wife, Agnes Collins. Mrs. Hunter returned to Raleigh with enough money from Collins and other benefactors to begin the construction of St. Agnes Hospital on St. Augustine's campus (Cobb, 1961).

St. Agnes Hospital and Training School for Colored Nurses opened on October 18, 1896, in a vacant house. There was a single cold-water faucet located in the kitchen. When hot water was needed for sterilizing, cooking, and other necessities, it was heated on a wood stove and carried in buckets to where it was needed. The hospital laundry consisted of three washtubs and a large iron kettle in the front yard. Obtaining ice required a four-mile trip by horse and buggy to downtown Raleigh. There were no screens on the windows, and heat was supplied by burning wood, while light was obtained from oil lamps. The administrative office was a multipurpose space that also served as a reception area, dining room, surgeon's dressing room, and occasionally as the morgue (Halliburton, 1937). The hospital opened with great fanfare, but in the first week, no patients came for care. During the second week, a man with typhoid fever was admitted and quickly recovered. Within six months, 16 inpatients and 35 dispensary or outpatients were treated. In addition, 223 people received medical and nursing care in their homes from St. Agnes' Hospital personnel. The first baby born at the hospital was appropriately named Agnes by her parents, Mr. and Mrs. Griffin. Agnes Griffin went on to become a prominent physician practicing for decades in New York City (Halliburton, 1937). From the beginning, St. Agnes had duel missions: to offer health care for local residents and to provide nurses training for interested students. On October 18, 1896, the first four student nurses were admitted and were taught by a faculty of eight. In 1898, St. Agnes graduated its first two nurses, Anna Augusta Groves and Effie Wortham, both of Raleigh (Pollitt, 2014). Between 1898 and its closure in 1961, approximately 500 nurses graduated from St. Agnes Hospital School of Nursing and gave untold hours of care to some of the poorest and most vulnerable citizens across North Carolina and the globe (Cobb, 1961).

A report from 1898 demonstrated that the hospital had become a vital part of Raleigh's African American community. During that year, 60 people were treated inside the hospital, and 23 operations were performed. These patients received a total of 1,670 days of care. An additional 436 people were treated through the dispensary/clinic (Halliburton, 1937). A 1904 fire necessitated the construction of a new hospital to replace the old wooden building. St. Augustine students quarried most of the stone and provided most of the labor to erect the new four-story, 75-bed St. Agnes Hospital. The stone hospital was completed, and patients were admitted in 1909. Demand for the hospital's services increased in the summer of 1916 when Shaw University administrators

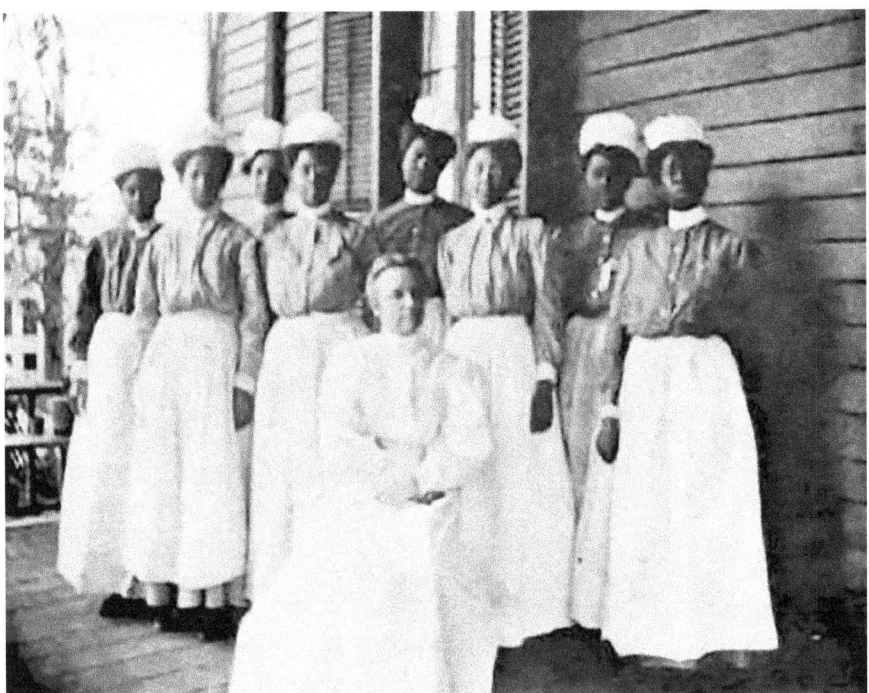

Nursing students and teacher at St. Agnes Hospital, Raleigh, ca. 1890. In Hartshorn and Penniman 1910.

closed Leonard Hospital, leaving St. Agnes as the only African American hospital in the capital city (Cobb, 1961).

On December 17, 1926, the hospital suffered another major fire. Patients were transferred to the McCauley Private Hospital in Raleigh, as St. Agnes Hospital was devastated and unusable. A fundraising campaign ensued to raise enough money for the hospital's rebuilding and expansion, as well as to add a sprinkler system to reduce the risk of future fires ("The McCauley Private Hospital," 1927). Probably the most unexpected donors to the rebuilding campaign were members of the Raleigh Ku Klux Klan. At the first meeting of the fundraising committee in 1922, three members of the Raleigh Klan chapter appeared in full regalia of robes and hoods. They handed a letter and five $10.00 bills to the Rev. Milton Barker who was chairing the meeting. The letter read:

> Dear Sir, Believing in the sincerity of the movement and being in sympathy with the furthering of such a worthy and beneficent cause, the Klan hereby declares

it's interest in the success and future of St. Agnes Hospital for colored people and hereby makes known its desire and willingness to lend support. It gives great pleasure, therefore, at this opportunity to tender, as a visible sign, the pledge of the Raleigh Klan to this cause, written for the sum of $100.00 dollars. And enclosed herewith are (5) $10.00 as the first payment on this pledge with the hope of the Klan for the great success of the campaign ["Raleigh Ku Klux Klan," 1922, p. 2].

The donation from the Klan, symbolic of the local white support for St. Agnes Hospital, was joined by donations from the white Raleigh Red Cross, Kiwanis Club, Rotary Club as well as individual donations ("Rotarians endorse," 1922, p. 10). *The Raleigh Times* editorialized:

"I don't know of an institution in the South that does more for the poor," Dr. John McKee City Physician said on Saturday. "The patients get good nursing and medical attention regardless of the fee. The hospital does an untold amount of good. The City could ill afford to get along without St. Agnes" ["St. Agnes Hospital," 1926, p. 8].

Of the $43,071.72 dollars raised, $25,371 came from African Americans and $17,751 came from white supporters. The restoration of the hospital was soon underway, and by the end of the school year it was complete. The new building ushered in a period of achievement at St. Agnes Hospital and School of Nursing. Demand for St. Agnes Hospital's beds and home care from its nursing students and staff was high. The hospital was experiencing great success. However, it did not last long. The stock market crash of 1929 and resulting Great Depression created many financial hardships for the hospital and school of nursing (Boykin, 1966). Many humanitarian organizations providing health and educational services for disadvantaged people were forced to close.

St. Agnes Hospital and School of Nursing, while remaining open, suffered in a variety of ways. Enrollment dropped to only 17 nursing students as potential students delayed their educations to earn money to keep family members fed and younger siblings in school (*St. Agnes Record*, 1932). As enrollment declined, fewer dollars were available for faculty salaries. Additionally, many patients were unable to pay for their care, even at the low rate of a dollar a day for a bed in a ward and three dollars a day for a private or semi-private room. The semi-private rate covered a room fee as well as meals, medications, dressings and nursing care.

In 1930, St. Agnes provided 20,235 days of patient care at an average per diem cost of $ 1.91. These figures do not include 3,158 days of care for expectant mothers who could work in non-professional jobs at the hospital for three months in lieu of paying for labor, delivery and newborn care (Halliburton, 1937). As the Great Depression continued through the 1930s, longtime supporters of St. Augustine University and St. Agnes Hospital could no longer contribute as much or as often as they used to, decimating the operating budgets of both institutions (Boykin, 1966). Conditions at St. Agnes Hospital were echoed in many African American hospitals across the state.

The plight of St. Agnes Hospital during the years of the Great Depression was chronicled in the *St. Augustine Record*, a quarterly newsletter that was sent to alumni and friends of the school. The following excerpts reflect the difficult days that the hospital faced in the early 1930s:

> There seems but little to write of St. Agnes Hospital since all our efforts are directed towards keeping open in order to minister to a people who have but little for food and nothing for hospitals or doctors [St. Agnes Hospital, 1931, p. 1].
>
> The present buildings (of St. Agnes Hospital) have room for one hundred patients, for the most part charity cases. The low prices paid for cotton and tobacco have made it almost impossible for the patients to pay for hospitalizations.... In spite of our poverty we have managed to keep open and no one needing care has been turned away from the door because of our lack of funds [St. Agnes Hospital, 1932, p. 2].
>
> There seems little to record that is new about St. Agnes Hospital since the struggle to economize more and more in the use of supplies and to limit purchases to the absolute necessities are the same things most institutions are doing [St. Agnes Hospital, 1933, p. 2]

Despite these trying circumstances, St. Agnes Hospital and School of Nursing continued to provide care and educate nursing students and medical interns. Between 1932 and 1954, approximately 80 physicians received advanced training at St. Agnes Hospital (Cobb, 1961). The hospital was accredited by the American Medical Association and the American College of Surgeons for training interns and residents in medicine, surgery, obstetrics, and gynecology (Delany, 1930).

The good works and reputation of St. Agnes Hospital resulted in sizable donations from the city of Raleigh, the Duke Endowment, the Protestant Episcopal Church, the American Church Institute for Negroes, and the Julian Rosenwald fund. These monies along with hard work, professional dedication and prayer kept St. Agnes Hospital open during the darkest days of the Great Depression (Halliburton, 1937; Ross, 1932).

By the mid–1950s, in order to keep up with advances in medical, surgical and obstetrical care, St. Agnes needed more funding than could be found by leaders of the Episcopal Church or of St. Augustine College. The various philanthropies that had contributed steadily in the earlier years could not commit to the sums necessary to bring St. Agnes Hospital in line with current hospital accreditation standards. At the same time, Wake County, with a population approaching 170,000, was home to several private white hospitals as well as St. Agnes, but had no public hospital. The private hospitals founded between 1878 and 1920 all needed extensive renovation to provide state-of-the-art care. In 1955, Wake County voters approved a $5 million bond issue to build a new 380-bed Wake Memorial Hospital as well as four 20-bed hospitals in Wake Forest, Apex, Zebulon and Fuquay-Varina ("A bit of history," 2014). Wake Memorial Hospital opened in 1961 with racially segregated wards, but all citizens of Wake County were admitted for care. Further, all eight African American physicians in Wake County had staff privileges in the Negro wards (Cobb, 1961). St. Agnes Hospital closed shortly after Wake Memorial Hospital opened. The stone shell of the building still sits on the St. Augustine University campus as a visual reminder of the care and education provided to thousands of African Americans during the Jim Crow era.

McCauley Private Hospital

Dr. Lewyn Eugene McCauley was born on January 28, 1883, to Roger E. and Martha A. McCauley in Wilmington, North Carolina. He was the oldest of six children, having five younger sisters. McCauley graduated from Kittrell College in Kittrell, North Carolina, in 1901 and from Leonard Medical School (LMS) in Raleigh in 1905. After graduating from LMS, Dr. McCauley spent a year in post graduate studies at the University of Pennsylvania, followed by two years teaching at his alma mater. Later, he did more port-graduate work at Freedmen's Hospital in Washington, D.C., and St. Phillips Hospital in Richmond, Virginia ("The old-timers page," 1954). Next, he joined the medical staff at St. Agnes Hospital where he provided patient care, as well as instruction in the nursing school (Sammons, 1990).

The first newspaper announcement of Dr. McCauley's plans to open a hospital appeared on January 13, 1916, in the *New York Age*. In an article titled "Raleigh to have a colored hospital," readers learned that Dr. Lewyn McCauley and Dr. F.J. Thorton were collaborating on a hospital that would be "strictly under the management of colored physicians" (1916, p. 1). Several years passed before this idea became a reality.

On June 23, 1923, Dr. McCauley opened the McCauley Private Hospital (MPH) at 513 S. Wilmington Street in Raleigh, where he specialized in surgical care of women and infants. The hospital was a brick building with 12 beds and 3 bassinets ("Private hospital," 1923). It was the only private African American hospital to be given a Class "A" rating from the American Hospital Association ("Association recognizes," 1942). Drs. Rufus Samuel Vass, Peter F. Roberts, and Golan S. Perry, all of whom were on the medical staff and nursing instructors at the St. Agnes Hospital, joined him in his new endeavor (Fisher & Douglas, 2015). Some of the nurses who worked in the hospital were Alice Hall, Madge Jeflers, Luvenia Jones, Madeline Richardson, Elina D. Taylor, Dancy Taylor, Anna B. Wingfield, Dorothy Brinson, and Versie Hobbs. After only two months of operation, the *New York Age* published this report:

> The McCauley Private Hospital located at 513 South Wilmington Street, Raleigh, NC is proving itself a great help to Raleigh people and those of nearby towns. This institution is meriting for itself more and more praise each day on account of the wonderful work being done there for the patients admitted. The people are proud of this institution both from the stand point of service as well as its low mortality rate. Since the opening of this hospital in the latter part of June, there has occurred only one death; the institution having been practically full since opening. The place is kept scrupulously clean, is comfortable and cheerful. We wish to congratulate Dr. McCauley in establishing such a place for his people. A place of this kind has been long wanted and needed by the people. Dr. McCauley is proving that the colored man can establish, maintain, manage and control responsible institutions creditably ["Raleigh, NC," 1923, p. 5].

While MPH generally served African Americans who could afford a private hospital and had obstetrical, gynecological, and/or pediatric health problems, the hospital and its staff also served the wider community in times of need. In 1927, St. Agnes Hospital suffered a devastating fire that caused all of the patients to be relocated. Dr. McCauley accommodated as many of the sickest patients as his hospital could hold and continued to admit many charity patients until St. Agnes could be rebuilt ("The McCauley Private Hospital," 1927).

An article in the *New York Age* from June 20, 1925, mentions Dr. McCauley and his hospital, noting:

> Among the outstanding features of the meeting [of the piedmont Chapter of the Old North State Medical Society] was the surgical clinic conducted by Dr. L.E. McCauley of Raleigh. Dr. McCauley is one of the leading surgeons of the South. He owns and conducts the McCauley Private Hospital at Raleigh, one of the leading hospitals of its kind in the State. During the time since it was first established, just a little less than two years ago, he has handled nearly 500 operative cases with an exceeding degree of success. Dr. McCauley specializes in gynecology, and during this meeting demonstrated some very scientific procedures to the men who were present ["Raleigh," 1925, p. 9].

By the 1940s, the hospital was "equipped with many of the latest medical facilities. One of the features of the plant is a well-lighted Operating Room and a modern x-ray machine" ("Association recognizes," 1942, p. 10). Due to the costs of maintaining the hospital's well-trained staff and up-to-date equipment, MPH could only afford to admit self-paying patients unless in exceptional circumstances. Because of the limited number of affluent African Americans, the facility remained small.

From 1927 through 1939, Dr. McCauley operated a nursing school at the hospital. In 1940, the North Carolina Board of Nursing required that student nurses train in a facility with an average daily census of 50 patients. McCauley and his colleagues could not meet that standard, so the nursing school closed. The hospital continued providing vital care to the community through the years of the Great Depression and World War II (State Archives, 2016; "Raleigh hospital marks," 1948). In 1954, the hospital recorded 1,029 days of patient care. By the middle of the 20th century, Raleigh's hospitals, both white and African American, were showing their age. Rex Hospital, a predominantly white facility, opened in 1894, St. Agnes Hospital was founded in 1896, the white Mary Elizabeth Hospital was erected in 1911, and McCauley Private Hospital followed in 1923. In 1955, the voters of Wake County passed a bond issue to construct a modern hospital that would be open to all, although there would be segregated wings for white and African American patients. In 1961, the new Wake County Memorial Hospital admitted it first patients, and the owners and administrators of the other hospitals began closing their facilities (Johnson & Murray, 2008). Dr. McCauley was 76 years old when Wake County Memorial Hospital (now Wake Medical Center) opened. He died there the next year, on March 18, 1962, of an abdominal blockage ("Dr. L. McCauley," 1962).

Throughout his life, Dr. McCauley was active in and led many social, political, religious, and professional organizations in Raleigh,

North Carolina, and across the country. He served as President of the Raleigh chapter and then the statewide Old North State Medical Society. He was chairman of the surgical section of the National Medical Association and Director of the Farmers and Merchants Bank in Raleigh; Master Mason; served on the Board of Trustees of Kittrell College; was President of the Raleigh chapter of the NAACP; a director of the Richard Harrison Library, a director of the African American Raleigh YMCA, and held various offices in the Elks, Knights of Pythias, Phi Beta Sigma fraternity, and the Raleigh Interracial Commission. In addition to his civic and professional involvement, Dr. McCauley was active in the African Methodist Episcopal Church, teaching Sunday school and serving on the Board of Directors (Yenser, 1942; Fisher & Douglas, 2015). In 1952, the Raleigh Masonic Kabala Temple selected Dr. McCauley as "Citizen of the Year." A *Carolina Times* editorial on April 5, 1952, praised his selection:

> The recent selection of Dr. L. E. McCauley of Raleigh as the "Citizen of the Year" by Kabala Shrine Temple is an honor well deserved by the noted physician whose service to his race, as a churchman, civic, business and fraternal leader, as well as a doctor, spans nearly a half century. In honoring Dr. McCauley, Kabala Temple has honored itself. The example set by the Raleigh physician deserves careful scrutiny by the younger men of the profession, who are to a great extent so elusive in their attitude that they could be easily classed as downright selfish. One only needs to look around him in the direction of the church, civic, business and social life of the average community to discern that a majority of the younger Negro physicians make little or no contributions, financially or otherwise to the struggles of the race other than the practice of their profession. The record shows that Dr. McCauley has served his people in most every field of endeavor in which they are engaged. For a long number of years he has served freely on the boards of church, business, social and fraternal organizations. Not only has he given of his time, energy and advice, but he has put his money in them as well. The CAROLINA TIMES felicitates the Kabala Temple for its selection of Dr. McCauley as the 1951 "Citizen of the Year." It is our honest belief that there is no other physician of the State who is more deserving of the honor than this polished gentleman of the medical profession who has wrought so well in the city of Raleigh ["A well-deserved Honor," 1952, p. 2].

Over half a century has passed since Leonard Hospital, St. Agnes Hospital, or McCauley Private Hospital admitted patients. Their very existence is largely forgotten. However, these institutions provided high-quality medical care for thousands of people in times of pain and crisis. In addition, they taught the first African American physicians and nurses in North Carolina, then launched them across the state and around the globe to build other hospitals and nursing schools while working to heal some of the world's most vulnerable people.

Charlotte, Mecklenburg County

The first known inhabitants of the region that is now Mecklenburg County were the Catawba people. In the mid–1700s, Europeans, primarily Scottish Presbyterians and German Lutherans, and enslaved Africans took over large swaths of Catawba lands. University of North Carolina at Charlotte history professor Dr. Dan Morrill (2001) writes about this transition:

> By the 1760s, after only a decade of persistent white occupation, much of the Catawba's lands had been sold, bartered, or lost. The Catawba nation had dwindled to a population of about 1000, for in addition to tribal warfare they suffered from contact with European diseases and vices: chiefly smallpox and whiskey [p. 5].

On the eve of the Civil War, approximately a third of the residents of Mecklenburg County were enslaved. Of the total population of 17,374, 10,543 were white, 6,541 were enslaved and 290 free African Americans. At that time, Charlotte was a small trading center that served surrounding farms and plantations. The town grew with the arrival of the railroad in the 1850s. After the Civil War, the local economy, built on slavery, collapsed. Charlotte transitioned from an agricultural center to a hub of industrial development, primarily in textile production. By 1900, Charlotte had become an industrial and commercial center and North Carolina's largest city (Lunsford, 2013). In the decades around the turn of the 20th century, thousands of people escaped rural poverty to work in Charlotte's mills and factories. The population of Charlotte quintupled from 7,000 in 1880 to over 34,000 by 1910 (U.S. Census Bureau, 1880–1910). According to the 1920 U.S. Census, there were approximately 22,000 whites, 11,000 African Americans, and three Chinese residing in the city. In the late 19th and early 20th centuries, several general hospitals opened in Charlotte (Lunsford, 2013). The first was the white-only Charlotte Home and Hospital, which opened in 1876. Another decade would pass before African Americans in Charlotte received local hospital care.

The Union/Colored Hospital, 1887–1894

The first African American hospital in Charlotte opened in 1887 and was known by two names. The first was the Colored Hospital because the patient population was confined to African Americans, and the second was the Union Hospital, reflecting the cooperation between white and African American Charlotte-area women who founded the hospital. These women came to know each other while working in the temperance movement of the 1870s and 80s. In parallel organizations, African American and white Charlotte chapters of the Women's Christian Temperance Union coordinated efforts to prohibit alcohol sales in the area. Although the temperance movement was ultimately unsuccessful, in the mid–1880s, many of the women who were engaged in this movement took up the cause of establishing an African American hospital (Greenwood, 1994). Both groups, each working with members of its own race, raised funds, recruited physicians to volunteer their time, sought donations of supplies and equipment, and coordinated efforts to make the hospital a reality. On February 1, 1887, the Union/Colored Hospital (UCH), opened in a two-room rented house on Myers Street (Greenwood, 1994). The white female Board of Managers was composed of Mrs. R.D. Johnston, credited with founding the hospital, Mrs. Hirshinger, President, Mrs. Pitcher, Treasurer, Mrs. H.A. Deal, Secretary, and Mrs. Liddell, Mrs. R.M. White, Mrs. J.L. Morehead, Mrs. M.A. Osborne, and Mrs. Samuel Whittkoski ("Report of the Colored," 1887). African American women—including Mrs. W.W. Smith, Mrs. Robert Johnson, Mrs. Dick Pethel and Mary Lynch—were equally active in the hospital committee (Greenwood, 1994).

Infrequent items in local newspapers reported on the hospital's progress. The first, dated December 12, 1886, was an invitation to the public to attend an art exhibit staged to raise money in support of the hospital's opening ("Notice of art," 1886). This piece was followed four months later by a letter to the editor in the *Charlotte Observer* from the hospital's Board of Managers:

> The hospital was formally opened February 1rst for the reception of patients and since that time four women and two men have been treated by attending physicians.... Meals and medicines have been furnished to three persons outside the hospital, one of whom could not be admitted on account of contagious disease.... The washing for the hospital is attended to by the colored Women's Christian Temperance Union with no charge. Mrs. Eliza Morehead has been selected by the colored Women's Christian Temperance Union as matron, and it

gives the Board of Managers pleasure to say she has filled the position most acceptably ["Report," 1887, p. 4].

Dr. R.J. Brevard, a white physician, and Dr. T.J. Williams, an African American physician and member of the first graduating class at Leonard Medical School, volunteered their services.

Many of Charlotte's pharmacists agreed to significantly reduce the cost of medicine for patients in the UCH ("Hospital," 1887, p. 13). Several African American and white churches, individuals, and organizations donated money, furniture, and supplies to the hospital. Supporters outside the region sent barrels of used clothing and bedding items. In February 1887, the costs of rent, wages for the matron, medicines, food, wood for heating, and incidentals totaled $105 ("The hospital for colored," 1887). On February 1, 1888, the Board of Managers issued an annual report that foreshadowed the financial issues that would ultimately lead to the hospital's demise. They were worried about a "remarkable falling off" of donations and a "dwindling list of subscribers" ("Report," 1888, p. 4). The report, published in several local newspapers, ended by asking the general public for donations to the hospital. In addition to the general appeal, the hospital leaders' fundraising efforts included a benefit baseball game, a bazaar, a speaking tour, and a music concert ("Black Diamond Quartet," 1888; "A card of thanks," 1886; "An appeal for the colored hospital," 1891; "Charlotte Chronical," 1891). Individuals responded to the pleas for donations and sent goods and supplies to the hospital. A list of supporters and their gifts in 1888 included F.R. Durham who gave potatoes, R.B. Alexander who donated flour, G.M. Holobaugh's contribution was sweet potatoes, and both Mr. Mosteller and J. Hagler gave the hospital beef. Mrs. S.V. Young provided Thanksgiving dinner for the patients and staff ("The Colored Hospital," 1888).

The number of patients and hospital coffers grew as reflected in the title of the second annual report: *Excellent Showing for the Institution*. A total of 485 days of patient care were provided in the second year for a total cost of $240.14. No patients were billed for services ("The Colored Hospital," 1889). The increasing numbers of patients outgrew the facilities' ability to house them. The Board of Managers erected a larger building in September 1889, that was "sixty feet by thirty containing seven rooms of good size" ("An appeal," 1891, p. 4).

Mrs. Jane Wilkes, a white Charlotte community activist, led a second group of women who decided local African Americans needed a different hospital. Perhaps they were motivated by denominational rivalry. At least three white congregations in Charlotte built denomination-specific hospitals between 1876 and 1906. The Episcopalians established St. Peter's Hospital in 1876, the Presbyterians formed Presbyterian Hospital in 1903 and the Catholics built Mercy Hospital in 1906 (Long, 1972). Perhaps Wilkes and her group operated out of anti–Semitism since Mrs. Hirshinger, the founder of the UCH, was Jewish. For reasons that are not clear, instead of working with the women who founded the UCH, in the 1880s, Wilkes and her colleagues began raising money for the new Good Samaritan Hospital. The women who were running the UCH were unhappy with this development. In a letter to the editor of the *Charlotte News*, they wrote in part:

> That this work is suffering from lack of sympathy [money] ... is both palpable and peculiar. Some doubt the need for the facility. If there is a necessity for two [hospitals], there is a necessity for one and the work of establishing another has been convinced while the one already in operation and with constant demands upon its charity, is suffering from want of help ["A good work," 1889, p. 3].

Charlotte was unique in North Carolina in having two competing groups of women working to establish and maintain separate hospitals for African Americans in the same town at the same time. This caused confusion and split loyalties among African American hospital supporters, ultimately leading to one's demise. The women's committee supporting the UCH was an ecumenical, interracial coalition who primarily sought local support. The women backing the Good Samaritan Hospital were seven, Episcopalian, white women appointed by the Bishop of the Diocese. They primary sought donations from Episcopal women's organizations outside the south. The *Charlotte News* interviewed Wilkes about the two competing hospitals:

> The hospital about which Mrs. Bainbridge is to lecture ... is a wooden building containing only two or three rooms.... I have never been connected with it except as a subscriber and well-wisher. The one for which I have been working and collecting for years before the other was thought of, is the Good Samaritan Hospital ... it is a two story, brick, home with 8 rooms with closets, store rooms, and bathrooms.... For this hospital I have never yet asked aid in Charlotte. It has been built entirely by the generous gifts of Northern friends ["About the colored hospital," 1891, p. 1].

Four days after Wilkes' interview appeared in the newspaper, the Managers of the UCH issued a retort, reminding *Charlotte News* readers that they had already erected a seven-room building with closets, and that the facility had rarely been empty since its inception in 1887. They again asked for donations to offset a current debt of $200 ("An appeal," 1891). Both groups were initially successful in their fundraising efforts. In the days before any government programs paid for hospital construction or care, the costs of running a charity hospital were substantial.

The next article in the local newspapers appeared two years later in 1893. An item in the *Charlotte Observer* informed readers that the Board of Managers for the UCH was composed of "various Christian denominations and Hebrews, who have been assisted by members of the different churches of the colored people" ("The Board of Managers," 1893, p. 2). On December 23, 1893, UCH managers appealed to Charlotte residents to "give the inmates [patients] a share of their Christmas bounty" ("A card," 1893, p. 4). In 1893, the last year the UCH was open, 48 patients were admitted and 47 recovered ("The Union Hospital," 1894). Perhaps because the larger, more substantial Good Samaritan Hospital opened in 1891, donations to the UCH dropped precipitously. It closed in 1894, and its building became a school for African American children ("Training colored youth," 1895).

Good Samaritan Hospital and School of Nursing, 1891–1960

The Good Samaritan Hospital (GSH) was rooted in the compassion of a group of Charlotte area, white, former Confederate nurses led by Jane Renwick Smedburg Wilkes. After the Civil War, Wilkes and other former Confederate nurses formed the Ladies Hospital Association. In 1876, Wilkes was also President of the Women's Aid Society of St. Peter's Episcopal Church in Charlotte. In these capacities, she was a leader in the establishment of the first civilian hospital in North Carolina, the Charlotte Home and Hospital, soon renamed St. Peter's Hospital, which opened in 1876 (Huffman & Hatchett, 1985). By law and custom, St. Peter's Hospital and its School of Nursing were only open to whites. Although the Wilkes family had owned slaves before the Civil War and Jane's husband, John Wilkes, was a captain in the Confederate Army, Mrs. Wilkes advocated for a hospital to serve the needs of ill and injured African Americans in Charlotte and Mecklenburg County (Pollitt & Reese, 1999). Early documents from GSH described the living conditions of the African American people it hoped to serve. Their homes were described as "crowded and squalid," and they suffered from "poverty which bars them from food and medicine they need" ("Good Samaritan Hospital," 1892, p. 7). Greenwood (1994), discussed Wilkes' role in founding GSH:

> In 1882 veteran reformer Jane Wilkes Peter's Episcopal Church, began collecting funds from northern Episcopal congregations for a black hospital. In 1888, she had raised enough money to purchase a lot on Hill Street in the Third Ward, and in December, 1888, she had the cornerstone laid for the hospital. Three years later the hospital opened. Although the funds for establishing Good Samaritan seem to have come almost exclusively from whites, the black residents of Charlotte played a key role in administering the hospital [p. 111].

The laying of the cornerstone on December 18, 1888, was a major cause for celebration. According to a local newspaper, a procession left the African American St. Michael's Episcopal Church at 3:00 in the afternoon. It was led by a Masonic fraternity followed by clergy of both races. Next were the dignitaries of the city, including Dr. Mattoon, the President of the African American Biddle College (now Johnson C. Smith University), Mayor McDowell, and Captain and Mrs. Wilkes. The cornerstone was laid with full Masonic Rites. There were prayers and speeches welcoming the new hospital to the area ("The Good Samaritan," 1888; "Laying the cornerstone," 1888).

After three years of construction, the 20-bed GSH accepted its first patients on September 23, 1891. It was the third African American hospital to open in North Carolina, the first being Leonard Hospital in Raleigh and the second UCH of Charlotte. Frank Wilkes, son of hospital founder Jane Wilkes, described GSH's first patients in a 1939 article in *Southern Hospital*:

> The first patient entered under gruesome circumstances. He was found lying just inside the gate, unconscious, almost naked, and in the last stage of pneumonia. Those who brought him were evidently too frightened to knock at the door. His case was hopeless, but he had care and comfort in his last hours and a decent burial. The next patient, protesting and struggling violently, was brought in by two policemen. His doctor had advised his coming, and his family were willing, but he fought desperately against entering that strong place called a hospital where it was rumored people were sometimes carved up with butcher knives [p. 9].

The behaviors described in the quote are reflective of the fear many felt about the new institutions—hospitals. Most people's images of hospitalization probably came from Civil War era hospitals where amputations were the most commonly performed surgery. Over 60,000 soldiers lost a limb to an amputation from a Civil War surgeon. These surgeons were frequently referred to as "butchers" (Rutkow, 2005). Taking ailing family members out of the home and into the care of strangers was a foreign concept and behavior for people at the end of the 19th century.

The first report from the GSH covered the first seven months the hospital was in operation and showed six nurses provided 629 days of patient care for 12 patients. Like the women who ran the UCH, GSH Managers, with Wilkes as President, sought donations of money and goods to support the hospital. Their fundraising appeals noted, "It is a purely charity hospital, organized by charity to aid the poorest and most helpless class of people" ("Good Samaritan Hospital," 1892, p. 2). Donations in 1893 included boxes of clothing, ½ bushel of lawn seed, turnip seed, oysters, apples, quilts, 1 box of tobacco, and 1 box of soap ("Annual Report," 1893). A brief paper about Good Samaritan Hospital, written by Stewart Lillard (n.d.), a librarian at the University of North Carolina at Charlotte, described early donations to the hospital:

> In May of 1902, the Great American Tea Company donated ten pounds of coffee to the institution. Much financial support continued to come from the Woman's Auxiliary of several Episcopal dioceses—in New York, Massachusetts, Connecticut, New Jersey, and Washington, D.C. Additional support was generated from Charlotte's own black community—from the Colored Graded School, St. Michael's Parish Church, and from the Seventh Street Presbyterian Church [p. 2].

As noted earlier, the GSH Managers depended on Episcopalian groups from outside the south to support their endeavor. Although all African Americans were welcomes as patients, regardless of religious affiliation, donors were mostly Episcopalian, supporting a denomination enterprise.

The 1902 *Annual Report* of GSH describes the hospital's first building:

> The house is a two-story brick one, conveniently arranged with hot and cold water, and baths on each floor, large closets and store-rooms, four large rooms containing twelve beds for patients upstairs and downstairs reception and matron's rooms, kitchen, and rooms for nurse and servant. The house is well ventilated, cheerful and bright and well removed from neighboring houses as the lot is 100 feet by 200 feet, affording space for a good garden [p. 3].

The medical staff consisted on one white physician—Dr. Dennis O'Donoghue and two African American physicians—Dr. J.T. Williams—

Leonard Medical School class of 1896—and Dr. D. E. Caldwell, an 1890 graduate of the Leonard Medical School, soon followed by white physician J.W. Faison and African American physicians H.W. Pressley and M.T. Pope, a 1886 graduate of Leonard Medical School (Hoover & Lewis, 2009). All of the nursing staff were African American women, initially led by Charlotte Jackson, followed by Mrs. Anne Robinson Buchanan, RN (LaNey, 2000). A 1902 pamphlet titled "The churches work among the Negroes" described the 1899 patient population of GSH:

> 117 patients were admitted, a larger number than in any former year.... All kinds of cases were treated. Railroad, mine and machinery accidents, knife and gunshot wounds, diseases of the eye and throat, cancer, female diseases, besides many cases of typhoid fever and other ailments have tested the skill of surgeon and physician and the care of matron and nurses [p. 1].

A nursing school was added in 1903 with the first graduation in 1905. By 1920, it met all the North Carolina Board of Nursing standards, so its graduates could sit for the Registered Nurse Examination and become registered nurses (Rann, 1964).

During the 1920s and 1930s, with assistance from both the Duke Endowment and the Rosenwald Fund, the hospital continued to grow in services and size. In 1925, a 30-bed addition, the Jane Wilkes Memorial Annex, was erected. It contained an operating room and maternity ward. During 1930, the hospital cared for 927 patients, providing 8,641 bed care days at a daily per capita cost of $2.65. In that year there were 284 outpatient visits, 174 major surgeries, and 542 minor operations (Rice & Jones, 1994). The Duke Endowment covered most of the costs of the addition. Another fifty beds were added in 1937 for a total of 100 beds (Rann, 1964). Many professional, church, and civic organizations "adopted" a new patient room to furnish and decorate. Some of these organizations included the St. Martin's parish, the Knights of Pythias, and the Florence Nightingale Club, the professional association of African American registered nurses in Charlotte (Wilkes, 1939).

Within a decade, another fundraising effort was underway. A 1948 pamphlet titled "Be a good Samaritan" issued to educate potential donors about GSH reported that the hospital was approved by the American Hospital Association and the North Carolina Hospital Association and was seeking accreditation by the American College of Surgeons. The Nursing School was rated as Class A by the North Carolina

Board of Nursing and had an enrollment of 40 students. The medical staff consisted of 13 African American physicians and 118 white physicians, while the hospital employed 105 African Americans and three whites. There were 80 beds for adult patients, 12 for children, 20 bassinets in the newborn nursery, and an emergency room. GSH was seeking funds for two additional emergency rooms, a 30-bed addition for adult patients, and a new heating plant (Good Samaritan Hospital 1948).

In the 1950s, several factors contributed to the hospital's imminent closure. Advances in medicine and technology made the costs of equipping and staffing a modern hospital beyond the budget of the Protestant Episcopal Diocese of North Carolina. A Special Committee of the Diocese was formed to study this problem. Their May 1960 report reads in part:

> A consideration of the problems facing the Hospital of the Good Samaritan show clearly that hospital standards have changed, the expense of capital improvements have become enormous, and generally, are possible only through public funds ... the Trustees of the Diocese have certified ... that the continued operation of the trust as a hospital is impracticable [p. 1].

In addition to the financial difficulties the hospital faced, an incident in October 1959 abruptly shut down the nursing school. At that time, the hospital had a white administrator, Edward R. Frye. On October 8, nursing student Rubina Little of Thomasville posted a list of discriminatory practices at GSH. Frye immediately expelled her for this action. The next day, 22 nursing students went on strike to protest Little's expulsion, and they were indefinitely suspended ("Charlotte, N.C.," 1959). On Monday October 12, 1959, the Trustees of GSH met and backed Mr. Frye. The students refused to return to class, and the Hospital Executive Board abruptly closed the GSH School of Nursing on October 31, 1959 ("Hospital given," 1959). Without the nursing students to supplement the nursing staff, patient care suffered. The local National Association for the Advancement of Colored People (NAACP) demanded that GSH be closed and its patients transferred to the all-white, tax-supported Memorial Hospital (Lillard, n.d.).

Finally, even without financial problems and the closure of the nursing school, white-only, tax-supported hospitals were coming under increasing legal pressure to provide some care to African American taxpayers and their families. In 1961, the Episcopal Diocese of North Carolina deeded GSH to the City of Charlotte for one dollar. GSH was renamed Charlotte Community Hospital, and a successful local bond issue infused over a million dollars into hospital upgrades (Rann, 1964). Despite these improvements, Charlotte-area African Americans with some white supporters and help from the U.S. Department of Health, Education, and Welfare successfully agitated for an end to all racial discrimination at the all-white Charlotte Memorial Hospital. Dr. Reginald Hawkins, a Charlotte dentist and ordained minister, was one of these civil rights leaders. In March 1962, he led picketers at white-only hospitals in town, carrying signs with slogans including "The hospital is built on a rock of segregation" and "Is this a Christian tradition? Segregated hospitals?" (Shinn, 1962). Dr. Hawkins also held a prayer service on the lawn of Presbyterian Hospital imploring hospital officials to care for all people regardless of race (Rice & Jones, 1994). In 1963, administrators at all three white hospitals in Charlotte, under pressure from both local protesters and federal government officials in Washington, D.C., declared that all patients would receive equal treatment regardless of race (Cobb, 1964). Good Samaritan/Community Hospital continued to provide care for African American and white patients until 1982. It then functioned as the Magnolia Rest Home until 1990 when the city demolished the facility to make room for the Bank of America Stadium in downtown Charlotte (Campbell, 2016).

Patient Demographics for Selected Years, 1891–1901

Year	# of patients	Total "days of care"	# of self-pay patients	# of charity patients
9/23/1891– 5/10/1892	12	629	0	12
1894	54	1,402		
1899	117			
1900	108	1,365	30	78
1901	107	1,456	26	81

Source: Twelfth Annual Report, of the Good Samaritan Hospital (1903).

Southern Pines, Moore County

Pickford Sanitarium, 1896–1912

Moore County was initially home to Saura and Siouan Indians. Before the American Revolution, they were pushed off the land by immigrants from Germany, England, Scotland, and Ireland. Moore

County's population in 1860 was 11,427 of which 2,697 were African Americans made up of 2,513 enslaved people and 184 free African Americans (Moore County Heritage, 2005). The North Carolina economy was ravaged by the Civil War. By the 1870s, North Carolinians were struggling to find new ways to earn a living. While some turned to industrial development and textile mills, several Moore County residents founded health and golf resorts. Moore County, with towns including Southern Pines, Pinehurst, and Carthage, is situated in a part of southeastern North Carolina known as the sand hills (Moore County Heritage, 2005). This unique geological formation is a strip of ancient beach dunes that divide the Piedmont from the coastal plain. Because of the sandy soil, cotton and other commercial crops did not grow well in the area. The region did not prosper until the railroad arrived in the 1870s.

In the 1880s and 1890s, several health and golf resorts were developed in the sand hills, bringing wealthy white tourists to the area. Southern Pines, the first such resort, was founded by James T. Patrick in 1884. On 675 acres, he laid out a new town with ample housing and civic buildings. James Walker Tufts bought 6,000 acres nearby and created another new town, Pinehurst, in 1895. Unfortunately, neither town allowed African Americans to live within their boundaries (Moore County Heritage, 2005). Many African Americans worked as servants in resort hotels and private homes. The air in the sand hills is drier and warmer than much of the state. Many physicians at the turn of the 20th century thought that dry, pine-scented air was optimal for the treatment for tuberculosis, the second leading cause of death at that time (Moss, 2005). A quote from Dr. R.H. Lewis, Secretary of the North Carolina Board of Health in 1897, illustrates this assumption:

> in our long leaf-pine, sand-hill region, where the porous soil takes up the water so rapidly that one can walk dry-shod in a half-hour after the heaviest rain, it is dry enough for the consumptive, and yet he can enjoy the sight and smell of the "blessed rain from heaven," and be lulled to sleep by its patter on the roof [Lewis, 1897, pp. 18–19].

Around the turn of the 20th century, several sanitaria, specialized hospitals to treat tubercular patients, were set up in Eastern North Carolina to take advantage of these conditions. The only private facility to treat African American patients was the Pickford Sanitarium, established and owned by Dr. L.A. Scruggs, the first African American in North Carolina to establish a health care facility.

Dr. Andrew Lawson Scruggs, physician, pharmacist, and one of the first three African American physicians licensed by the state of North Carolina, was born a slave in Bedford County, Virginia, on January 15, 1857. After graduating from the Richmond Institute, he enrolled in Shaw University in Raleigh. He graduated first in his class in the Classical course and was simultaneously enrolled in the new Leonard Medical School. Scruggs graduated first in his medical school class in 1886 (Jones, Jones & Jones, 2004). In his valedictory speech he claimed, "The colored man must go forward, he must harness himself for battle, and we who stand before you tonight are pioneers of the medical profession of our race" (Scruggs, 1886, p. 3).

Shortly after graduation, Scruggs was appointed Resident Physician at Leonard Hospital, as well as lecturer in physiology, hygiene, and chemistry in the college department at Shaw, the first African American to hold these positions. In addition to his work at Leonard Hospital, Scruggs opened an office in Raleigh and began making house calls. He added to his workload in 1891, becoming the first African American campus physician and lecturer in physiology and hygiene at St. Augustine's University. When St. Agnes Hospital and School of Nursing opened on St. Augustine's campus in 1896, Scruggs was its first attending physician and lecturer (Murray, 1996). Scruggs was concerned about the number of people afflicted and dying from tuberculosis at a time when there were no sanatorium beds open to African Americans in North Carolina. He decided to open a sanitarium in Southern Pines (Hawkins, 2008).

Scruggs sought support for his new endeavor from Charles J. Pickford, a businessman from Massachusetts, the same benefactor who had supported him as

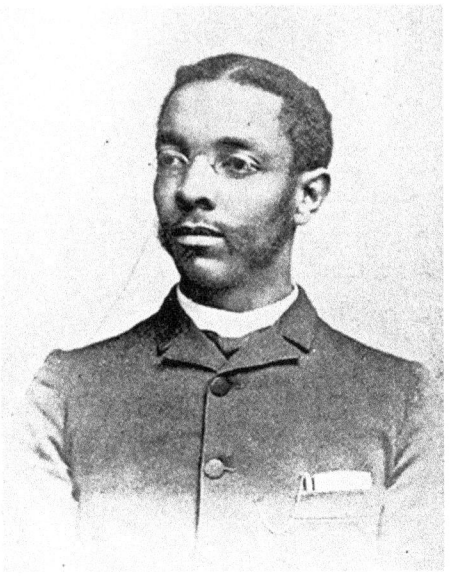

Dr. Lawson Andrew Scruggs graduated from Leonard Medical School in 1886. That same year he founded Pickford Tuberculosis Sanitarium in Southern Pines. In Scruggs 1893.

a student at the Richmond Institute. After Pickford's passing, his widow and daughter donated again to Dr. Scruggs' sanitarium, which bore the Pickford name. In 1897, the sanitarium received a charter from the North Carolina General Assembly, and in 1899, the General Assembly recognized the sanitarium as a charitable institution and endorsed its mission (Hawkins, 2008). In *The Southern Sanitarium* (1897), a journal written and edited by Dr. Scruggs, he described his plans to erect 16 pavilions (residence halls) to be built at a cost of $350 each and a central administration building that would cost $20,000.

The Ladies' Pickford Sanitarium Aid Society of Raleigh, an all–African American women's benevolent association, furnished the first residence hall. It was noted as "a fine building with sun parlors and ample piazzas has just been completed for the especial use of women" ("Conference," 1896, p. 34). By 1900, the Sanitarium also had a kitchen, dining room, nurses' department, offices, and three pavilions. The maximum capacity was 30 patients ("Conference," 1896). In February 1900, the new Hubbard building was dedicated with a ceremony of vocal and instrumental music and speeches. Supporters of the Pickford facility gave medicine, money, clothing, kitchen and office supplies, and other miscellaneous item ("Interesting exercises," 1900; Hawkins, 2008).

Pickford Sanatorium was open from December 1 through May 1 of each year and charged $15 a month. Treatments included rest, fresh air—sleeping on porches or with opened windows—a nutritious diet, and moderate activities for those recovering from the disease. To hasten recovery, expand lung function, and build muscle tone, patients were encouraged to work as gardeners on the Sanitarium's grounds, as carpenters on the facilities' buildings, and as printers of fundraising pamphlets, as well other jobs around the facility. According to Scruggs' own statistics, "Sixty-six percent of all patients that have been treated at Pickford Sanitarium have gone home relatively cured, and are now self-supporting" (Scruggs, 1901, p. 6). Acknowledging that even the most modern treatments often failed, Scruggs noted, "If we could not cure them we might give them comfortable quarters in which to die" (Scruggs, 1897, p. 12).

In every issue of the *Southern Sanitarium*, Scruggs listed needs for his sanitarium in a section titled "Our immediate needs" (Hawkins, 2008). In the March 1900 issue of the journal, he asked "for a nice little farm of ten acres, which will do much towards furnishing supplies for the Institution—vegetables, fruit for canning, milk, eggs, butter, chickens, etc." (Scruggs, 1900, p. 18–19). Scruggs also asked for a milk cow and a microscope (Hawkins, 2008).

Dr. Scruggs' accomplishments were numerous. He built the first African American sanitarium without denominational or significant philanthropic support. He willingly put his own health at risk to fight the scourge of tuberculosis when a cure was still elusive. He created and maintained a journal, the *Southern Sanitarium*, devoted to raise awareness and knowledge about the disease. Dr. Scruggs and his staff earned praise from newspapers as far away as Boston, as well as from a variety of organizations, such as the North Carolina Chamber of Commerce and the North Carolina House of Representatives. A very interesting editorial from *The Boston Transcript* was reprinted in the *Morning Post* of Raleigh on July 7, 1898. The editors noted that southern African Americans who had TB "often have far less care than is given a dog when sick in the North..." ("Substantial aid," 1898, p. 5). The editors went on to describe Dr. Scruggs and the Pickford Sanitarium: "He is a well-educated Negro physician and he has opened this convenient and well equipped home for invalids of his own race ... when I visited Southern Pines in March, there was an African prince among the patients" (p. 5).

Unfortunately, Pickford Sanitarium could not accept all of the people who applied to be patients at the institution. There were not enough beds, food, medicine, or staff to help all those who suffered. Despite donations from benefactors across the country and patient payments, the facility was continuously in financial trouble. Scruggs wrote in 1898: "The Nurse in Chief has been spending all the summer in Massachusetts and New York in the interest of the Sanitarium for consumptives.... The results have been very gratifying and she has made many friends for our work" (as cited in Hawkins, 2008, p. 39). In that same year, Dr. Scruggs gave up his private practice in Raleigh to spend more time fundraising for the Sanitarium. In the winter 1901 issue of *The Southern Sanitarian*, Dr. Scruggs pled for donations:

> Kindly therefore, help us by contributing 5c, 25c, 50c, $1.00 more or less, either in money or material supplies.... If after all, however, you find that you can do nothing, even then be kind enough to so write me and at the same time give us your sympathy and remember that
>
> > If you cannot give your thousands,
> > You can give your widow's mite,

All the least you do for Jesus,
Will be precious in his sight [Scruggs, 1901, p. 9].

Pickford Sanitarium operated for about 15 years, but the lack of finances needed to maintain the buildings, pay the staff, and provide food and medicine, along with Scruggs' declining health, forced the facility to close around 1912. Dr. Scruggs returned to Raleigh and died on December 1, 1914, at his home of nephritis at age 57 (Hawkins, 2008). Although some counties erected sanitaria with segregated wards for whites and African Americans, most North Carolina African Americans with tuberculosis would have to wait another 12 years for in-patient care. In 1924, the tax-supported North Carolina Sanitarium, which opened for white patients in 1908, opened a Negro Unit.

Durham, Durham County

Lincoln Hospital, 1901–1976

Durham County is located in the central piedmont of North Carolina. The land was originally home to Occaneechi and Eno Native Americans who were forced out by the 18th century to make way for German, English, Scotts-Irish, and other European settlers. Prior to the Civil War, most area residents were engaged in small-scale farming, while a few owned large plantations. About a third of the population in the area that would become Durham County, which formed in 1881, was African American. After the Civil War ended, tobacco became the primary cash crop with cigarette manufacturing and textile mills dominating the local economy (Anderson, 1990). The population in Durham County more than doubled in its early years from 18,000 in 1890 to 42,000 in 1920 ("Durham County," 2016). During this time, philanthropists established several hospitals in North Carolina, including Durham's Lincoln Hospital for African Americans.

In the late 1890s, after building a fortune from tobacco manufacturing, the Duke family, led by patriarch Washington Duke, considered building a monument to the enslaved people who remained loyal to their masters during the Civil War. Fortunately, Dr. Aaron McDuffie Moore, an 1888 graduate of the Leonard Medical School and the first African American physician to practice in Durham, and Mr. John

Merrick, Washington Duke's personal barber and founder of the North Carolina Mutual Life Insurance Company, convinced the Duke family to contribute their money to the establishment of an African American hospital instead of a monument. Watts Hospital, the only hospital in Durham at that time, did not accept African American patients, nor hire African American physicians or nurses (Watts & Scott, 1965).

The Dukes decided that a hospital was a suitable charity and donated $8,550 to the cause ("One Way," 1930). The cornerstone of the new Lincoln Hospital (LH) was laid at the intersection of Proctor Street and Cozart Avenue on July 4, 1901. Lincoln Hospital began admitting patients less than two months later. It was the fifth hospital for African Americans in North Carolina and the largest without a religious affiliation. Founded as a non-profit, general hospital, LH served all patients regardless of ability to pay. The hospital offered major and minor surgery, pediatric and obstetrical care, and a 24-hour emergency room.

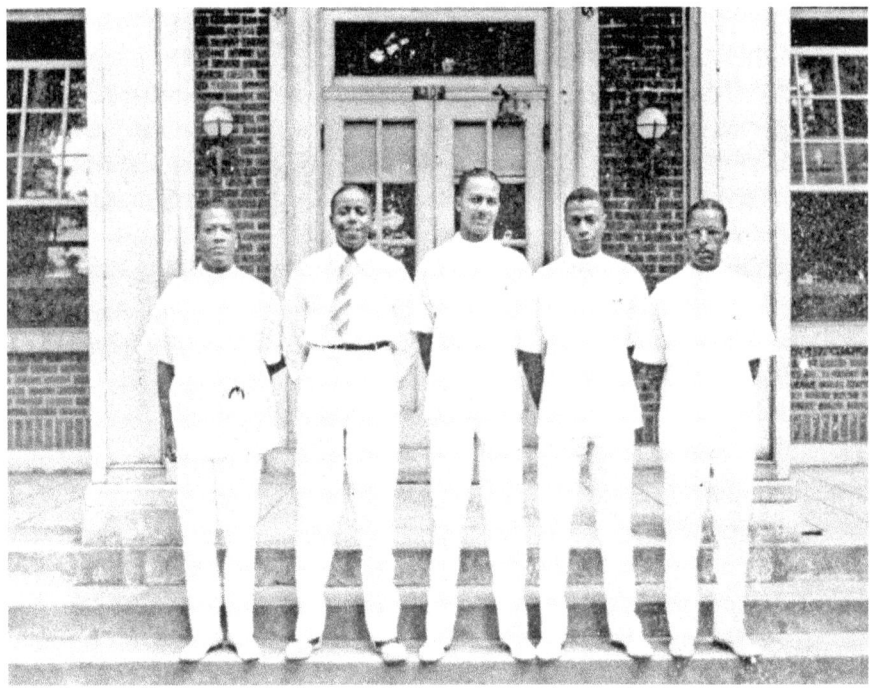

Resident staff, Lincoln Hospital, Durham, 1838–1839. Lincoln Hospital's 38th Annual Report, 1938.

It also maintained outpatient clinics for tuberculosis, cancer, and other adult medical issues. Early staff members included Dr. Moore, Superintendent, Dr. Stanford Lee Warren, an 1895 graduate of Leonard Medical School, and Dr. Charles H. Shepard, a 1901 graduate of Leonard Medical School as staff physicians, and Miss Julia Latta, a 1900 graduate of St. Agnes Hospital School of Nursing, as Nursing Superintendent (Reynolds, 2001). In keeping with the Duke's original intent, these words were inscribed at the entrance to the hospital: "With grateful appreciation and loving remembrance of the fidelity and faithfulness of the Negro slaves to the Mothers and Daughters of the Confederacy, during the Civil War, this institution was founded by one of the Fathers and Sons" (Brown, 2008, p. 5).

Nurse Latta was one of two original full-time employees when LH opened in 1901; the other was the janitor. In addition to her nursing duties, she did the hospital's laundry, cooking, and housekeeping. It quickly became apparent that the hospital needed more nurses, so when LH added a nurse training school in 1902, Nurse Latta added Nursing School Superintendent to her list of responsibilities (Reynolds, 2001). Under her leadership, 17 nurses graduated between 1905 and 1911. Nurse Latta left LH to become the first African American public health nurse in Durham County. Nurse Patty Carter replaced Miss Latta as the hospital's Superintendent of Nurses and the Superintendent of the nursing school. She remained in these positions for 24 years. Nurse Carter was a graduate of both the St. Agnes Hospital in Raleigh and Lincoln Hospital in New York City (Wicker, 2013).

As the years went by, demand for hospital services outpaced LH's physical facilities. From 1901 to 1925, 7,000 patients were admitted, most of them charity cases (Reynolds, 2001). A fire that decimated much of LH in 1924 served as a catalyst for the erection of a new brick building. The Duke family donated $75,000, the city and county governments jointly gave $25,000, and Durham's white and African American communities each raised about $25,000 for the new LH on Fayetteville Street. The fundraising figures demonstrate the spirit of racial cooperation in Durham in the 1920s (North Carolina Board, 1930). The new 87-bed hospital housed several specialty areas not found in the older wooden building. There was a dietetic lab for nurses training, an autopsy room, clinical laboratories, and an x-ray room (Wicker, 2013). In that same year, Benjamin Duke donated an additional

$25,000 for a nurse's dormitory. With the new facilities, LH was given an "A" rating by the North Carolina Board of Nursing.

In addition to the improved conditions for nurses and nursing education, LH also developed a partnership with Leonard Medical School to offer internships to medical school graduates. When Leonard closed in 1918, Lincoln established its own medical training programs. In 1925, LH was approved for intern training in the field of medicine by the Council on Medical Education and Hospitals, followed by approval for surgical internships by the American College of Surgeons in 1930 (Shepard, 1930). Twenty years later, LH earned full accreditation for a four-year surgery residency leading to board certification in 1950 (Watts & Scott, 1965).

North Carolina African American Hospitals with Internship and Residency Training Programs

Name of hospital	Internship/ Residency	Specialty areas	Years of existence
Leonard	Internship	Medicine	1912–1916
St. Agnes	Internship	Medicine, surgery, obstetrics/ gynecology	1914–1961
Lincoln	Internship/ Residency	Surgery	1925–1970s
Kate B. Reynolds	Internship Residency began in the 1940s	Medicine, surgery, obstetrics, pediatrics	Early 1940s– 1980s
Community	Residency	Medicine	1938–1967

Interns at Lincoln Hospital, 1925–1931

Name	Year
Russell Rice	1925
Enos S. Wright	1926
I.E. Turner	1926
Robert H. Green	1927
Leroy Hall	1927
G.E. Dudley	1928
R.M. Wyche	1928
G.E. Nightengale	1928
J.M. Dasher	1929
F.A. Moncur	1929
Floyd Green	1929
J.E. Alexander	1930

Name	Year
William Forrester	1930
A.B. Green	1930
William French	1931
Paul Cornely	1931
Alga Wade	1931

By 1930, the staff had grown to include five registered nurses, three interns, 35 nursing students, one orderly, two janitors, a fireman, and three cooks. Fifty-three physicians were admitting patients to the hospital ("One Way," 1930). The Duke Endowment and Rosenwald Fund contributed money to support salaries for supervising physicians in the 1930s to upgrade the skills of staff physicians and surgeons with the ultimate goal of improving patient care (Gamble, 1995). With the new facilities and additional staff, the quality and quantity of patient care increased. In 1925, 140 minor surgeries were performed. That number rose to 656 by 1930. In 1940, 1,399 minor surgeries and 236 major surgeries were performed, 21.502 laboratory tests were conducted, 1,796 x-rays were given, and a total of 20,858 days of care were provided to inpatients, while 5,636 people received outpatient care (Reynolds, 2001).

Beginning in the 1935, LH began to host annual continuing medical education conferences called the Lincoln Hospital Post-Graduates Clinic. Lincoln's proximity to the N.C. College for Negroes' dormitories, which provided housing for visiting physicians at a time when most southern hotels banned African Americans, made attending conferences in Durham much easier than many other North Carolina cities. The clinics drew African American physicians from North Carolina and neighboring states to hear speakers from the University of North Carolina at Chapel Hill, Duke University, and the State Board of Health (Ayanian, 1982).

Lincoln Hospital staff did their part to support the armed forces in World War II. At least two LH physicians served overseas, Dr. William A. Cleland and Dr. Robert Randolph. In addition, LH School of Nursing joined the U.S. Cadet Nurse Corps program, whereby students in the program received tuition, books, uniforms, and a stipend; in exchange, they were required to serve actively in essential civilian or federal government services for the duration of World War II (Reynolds, 2001). At the beginning of World War II, the U.S. Army Nurse Corps (USANC) did not allow African American nurses to join because of their race. As the need for more nurses became apparent, the Army dropped its ban in 1941. Nurse Della H. Raney Jackson, a 1937 graduate of LH, became the first African American Registered Nurse to enlist in the United States Army Nurses Corps (Pollitt, 2014). Registered Nurse Emma Lee Randolph, Operating Room Supervisor at LH also joined the UNANC during the War.

In 1950, Durham City and County government officials acquired Hill-Burton Act federal monies to expand both the African American Lincoln Hospital and the white Watts hospitals. A local bond measure passed as well, providing $333,700 to Lincoln and five times as much, $1.6 million, to Watts Hospital. Lincoln's local funding was matched with $258,700 in federal funds. These monies paid for the construction of a new 33-bed wing, completed in 1953, increasing the bed total at Lincoln to 123 (Anderson, 1990).

A 1961 article in the Durham-based *Carolina Times* titled "Lincoln Hospital linen day drive nets $481.90; Queen crowned" illustrates the great financial difficulties hospitals faced before the Medicare and Medicaid programs took effect in the late 1960s. The article describes the annual friendly competition Lincoln Hospital nurses entered seeking funds from their churches to purchase linens for the hospital. Whoever raised the most money was crowned "Miss Lincoln Hospital Linen Day." In 1961, Nurse Nettie Wilson won the contest by raising $110.05. During the celebration Mr. F.W. Scott, Lincoln Hospital administrator, noted:

> A patient doesn't realize that it takes numerous people to serve him. He only sees the nurse. He never sees the dietician. He doesn't realize that the cook, the laundry personal, the medical records librarian, lab technician, maintenance, administrative and clerical personal are all serving him. The patient doesn't really know what he's getting for his money. He has experts waiting on him and he gets all this for $23 a day ["Lincoln Hospital linen day," 1961, p. 3].

Despite the infusions of federal funds in the 1950s, both Lincoln and Watts Hospitals were outmoded facilities by the 1960s. A 1966 bond referendum to raise money to build a new, integrated Watts Hospital was soundly defeated by both whites and African Americans—by whites because they opposed integration and by African Americans because they did not want to lose Lincoln Hospital. Only two years later, a vote to fund a new, integrated Durham County General Hospital (DCGH), consolidating Watts and Lincoln hospitals in a new facility, passed overwhelmingly (Anderson, 1990). With Durham County General Hospital opening in 1976, Lincoln Hospital became a community health clinic and Watts Hospital was repurposed to house the North Carolina School for Science and Mathematics, a residential high school (Wicker, 2013).

Winston-Salem, Forsyth County

Forsyth County's first inhabitants are thought to be members of the Catawba and Keyauwee tribes (Merrell, 1989). In 1752, a group of Moravians settlers bought 99,000 acres in what is now Forsyth County and quickly created the towns of Bethania, Bethabara, and Salem as centers of religion and trade. In 1851, about a mile from the center of Salem, Winston, a more secular city, was officially established. In 1860, out of a total county population of 12,692, 1,784 were enslaved and another 211 were free African Americans (Hamrick, 2010). After the Civil War, the city of Winston quickly became a bustling industrial center. Tobacco magnate Richard Reynolds founded the R.J. Reynolds Tobacco Company. His company was one of the largest employers in the region. With increasing employment opportunities people from nearby rural areas moved into Winston and Salem for jobs. The African American population of Forsyth County rose from 15 percent at the start of the Civil War to almost 30 percent by 1900 (Bricker, 2008).

At the turn of the 20th century, the towns of Winston and Salem in central North Carolina had not yet merged but both supported the Twin Cities Hospital, where white residents of the towns were welcome for medical and surgical care and for hospital deliveries. However, as Prichard (1976) noted in the Winston-Salem area at the turn of the 20th century, "African Americans were cared for at home or not at all" (p. 246). Several North Carolina cities, including Charlotte, Durham, Raleigh, and Wilmington, relied on one major African American hospital in each community for decades. The history of African American hospitals in Winston-Salem, however, is composed of a series of hospitals opening and closing in fits and starts.

The first hospital, Slater, owes its origins to Simon Green Atkins and R.J. Reynolds. On June 11, 1862, Atkins was born into slavery in Chatham County, North Carolina. After graduating from St. Augustine University in Raleigh in 1880, he began his teaching career in his home county. After several years, Atkins decided to go to an educationally underserved area and start a new school. In 1892, using monies from the Slater Fund, a philanthropy founded by a northern industrialist, he established the Slater Industrial Academy in Winston, North Carolina, now known as Winston-Salem State University (Rauhauser-Smith, 2015). The school offered a classical education and a variety of vocational programs.

By the turn of the 20th century, Atkins and other school officials wanted to add a hospital and nursing school to the campus. At the same time, tobacconist R.J. Reynolds wanted a facility to treat his ill and injured African American employees. After a successful fundraising campaign, in which Reynolds matched the total amount of all other donations, the hospital and nurse training program opened on May 14, 1902 (Prichard, 1976). Atkins named the new hospital Slater Hospital in honor of the school's benefactor (Cue & Davis, 2000). The first three physicians to work at Slater Hospital were Dr. Frank S. Hargrave, a 1901 graduate of Leonard Medical School, Dr. John W. Jones an 1891 graduate of Leonard Medical School and Dr. H. Humphrey Hall, an 1887 graduate of Leonard Medial School ("Slater Normal School," 1903). During the first year, the hospital physicians treated 90 patients and performed 21 operations (Prichard, 1976). Lula C. Hairston, an 1896 alumna of the Slater Institute, graduated from the Freedmen's Hospital School of Nursing in Washington, D.C., in 1899. Upon her graduation, she returned to Slater Institute as the school's nurse, taking care of student health needs. When the hospital opened in 1902, Hairston became the Nursing Superintendent of the hospital and the director of the nurse training school. The nursing school was small, usually only two or three students were enrolled in the program (Report of the Commissioner, 1907). Graduates of the nursing program included Mary Montgomery Enloe ("Death," 1918) and Dorothy Hemphill Crawford ("Widely known," 1947). Two nurses, the nursing students, and the Ladies Auxiliary (composed of local women) cared for the patients who filled the hospital's 20 beds. Fees were $2 a week for care in a ward and $4 a week for care in a private bed. Many of the patients were indigent and unable to pay for their hospital care ("Slater Hospital," 2016). Nurse Hairston asked for donations of "anything in the line of medicine, hospital supplies and food" (Hairston, 1903, p. 37).

One of the duties of Nursing Superintendent Hairston was to solicit funds for the hospital. A successful fundraising event occurred on July 6, 1903, when she arranged an evening of "choruses, solos, recitations and pantomimes" at the African American Moravian Church, collecting about $25 for the hospital ("Successful entertainment," 1903). After the first year of operations, the hospital was $200 in debt (Prichard, 1976). A 1904 article in the *Winston-Salem Journal* demonstrates deep community support for the hospital:

> The ministers of the different churches have taken up several collections for the hospital which were very gratifying. Many useful articles and delicate foods necessary to the nourishment of the patients have been contributed. Several of the secret orders have sent to the hospital large collections of supplies. All winter the hospital has been full and the workers taxed to their uttermost. These expressions of interest however, have encouraged them in their work ["Great Interest," 1904, p. 1].

In April 1905, the great African American educator and founder of the Tuskegee Institute, Booker T. Washington, came to Winston-Salem to give a fundraising speech for Slater Hospital. About 800 people, of both races, attended his speech, each paying a dollar with some giving additional donations. Almost $1,000 was raised for the hospital's needed improvements and supplies.

In addition to financial difficulties, Slater Hospital was plagued with the lack of an adequate water supply. The hospital closed for several months when a well failed in the summer of 1904. The hospital then reopened on April 3, 1905, after a pipeline from the Salem water supply brought fresh water to the hospital ("Professor Washington," 1905). A report from the North Carolina Board of Public Charities (1906) shows Slater Hospital treated 53 patients in the seven months between April 3, 1905, and October 31, 1905. Of those, 28 were discharged, 10 died, and 15 remained in the hospital at the time the report was written. The hospital charged two to three dollars a week for care in the ward or four to six dollars for care in private rooms. Major operations cost $5 and minor procedures $2.50. The hospital also treated individuals who were unable to afford the care, including 35 charity patients, or about half, of the total admitted. In the early 1900s, the hospital grew to 25 beds with a staff of three to four nurses. Dr. A.J. Brown, Superintendent of Slater Hospital, noted a need for "a heating plant for the whole building, conveniences for the operating room, instruments and bedding" (North Carolina Board, 1906, p. 74).

In 1905, Mrs. Hunter, the Superintendent of St. Agnes Hospital, asked each of the nurses who had graduated from her program to write about their careers so she could put together a booklet for the St. Agnes Hospital's 10th anniversary. Nurse Nina E. Peoples, a 1904 graduate of St. Agnes Hospital School of Nursing, sent Mrs. Hunter an interesting letter, dated December 6, 1905, about Slater Hospital. Nurse Peoples moved to Winston in August 1905 to become head nurse at the hospital:

> I found three patients here and two junior nurses. I have admitted thirty-eight patients since August 28th. I have five patients now. The hospital is not in connection with Slater School now as it was from the first, but a separate institution. I have been the means for organizing four Ladies Hospital Clubs since coming here and the people are donating liberally to the support of the institution. The building is a two story wooden structure. On the first floor is an office; on right of entrance the Men's Ward with six beds; following patients' bath room with private ward number two; next nurses' dining room, next kitchen; a nice wide porch on the back. A porch running across the front completes the first floor with a gracious hall. On second floor there are seven rooms which are used for nurses and help with the exception of two. One is the linen room, the other private room number 3. The laundry is in the basement under the back porch. The site is beautiful, with a nice lawn surrounding the building [Peoples, 1905].

Slater Hospital continued to struggle financially. An April 30, 1909, article in the *Western Sentinel* reported that the Slater Hospital building was closed for an overhaul and would be ready for patients the next day, May 1, 1909 ("Slater Hospital," 1909). Just a few months later, in August 1909, an item appeared in the same newspaper stating: "We are glad to inform our friends that the Slater Hospital is again open and we think now under such an arrangement as will keep it open" ("Tag day," 1909, p. 2). However, a November 1910 report on the recent Winston Board of Aldermen meeting chronicles the continuing financial hardships Slater Hospital faced: "Dr. J.E. Dowdy, city physician stated to the board that the Slater Hospital had closed and that there was no place at the present time to take emergency cases for the colored people ... he stated the nurse at Slater Hospital had not been paid her salary in four months" ("Slater Hospital closed," 1910, p. 1).

Another article appeared in the March 1911 *Western Sentinel*, titled "Slater Hospital re-opened." Ultimately, the financial difficulties proved too much to overcome, and Slater Hospital closed for the last time in 1912. By that time, City Hospital, the local white hospital, had added a few beds for African Americans. The Slater Hospital building became a dormitory for Slater Institute. Slater Hospital's supporters continued to struggle to create a hospital for African Americans in Winston-Salem for decades (Prichard, 1976).

Williamson's Sanitarium

The closing of Slater Hospital was a great loss to the African American people of Winston-Salem. It did not take long for Dr. John C. Williamson, a 1913 graduate of Leonard Medical School, to open a sanatorium in Winston-Salem. An article in the June 7, 1914, *Winston-Salem Journal* reports:

> Dr. J.C. Williamson, colored, a former student of Slater school and graduate of Leonard Medical School and formerly a resident physician in St. Agnes Hospital, has opened up a private sanitarium for the colored people of the city at 831 Ida Bell Avenue Columbia Heights. He purchased the boys dormitory [most likely the former Slater Hospital building] and has thoroughly renovated it and made many improvements, converting it into an up-to-date hospital with accommodations for 10 patients. The paintings, decorations and excellent lighting of the rooms make them especially cheerful for the sick, and this institution is destined to prove of great benefit to the colored people of the city. It is thoroughly equipped with trained nurses and Dr. Williamson frequently furnishes nurses to the city physicians both white and colored. He is also conducting a small dispensary for the benefit of the hospital and the accommodation of the people living in the district. Dr. Williamson has been practicing in the city a little more than a year and is doing well. He is building up a larger practice and is considered one of the most promising graduates of Slater school ["Sanitarium for colored people," 1914, p. 7].

According to the 1917 North Carolina Board of Public Charities Report, Dr. Williamson's Sanitarium was a strictly private institution, admitting no charity cases. Dr. Williamson treated people with medical and surgical problems, as well as crippled children. Twenty-three patients were admitted in 1916. Of those, 16 were cured, one died, and six were still hospitalized at the time of the report. No records have been found detailing events at the Williamson Sanitarium after 1916. Because there were no denominational or philanthropic backers, there was no need for the annual reports and record keeping some other African American hospitals produced. Apparently, after 1916, African Americans in Forsyth County were again without a facility in which they could be treated by physicians and nurses of their own race. An item in the October 20, 1916, Twin City Sentinel reported that a committee of three physicians, Drs. A.H. Ray, John R. Henry, and Williams, from the Twin City Medical Society, the local African American association of physicians, pharmacists and dentists, were appointed to select a site for an African American Hospital (Colored doctors, 1916).

Ray's Hospital (aka Wray's Hospital)

Dr. Alexander Hamilton Ray, a 1908 graduate of Leonard Medical School, opened a 15- to 20-bed hospital at Thirteenth and Ridge streets around 1920. The building was a one-story wood frame home owned by his wife (Grimes, 1972). Ray's Hospital was listed in the city directories from 1920 to 1926 with Miss Lillian Northern as the nursing superintendent. According to Dr. Ray's obituary, over 600 operations were performed there ("Dr. A.H. Ray," 1954). A fire caused massive damage to the building in 1922, but Dr. Ray kept the hospital open. There are no available records explaining the reasons the hospital closed. Dr. Ray became the first physician for the students and staff at Winston Salem State University and remained in that position for over 25 years. The student health center is named in his honor.

After Ray's Hospital closed around 1926, African Americans in Winston-Salem needing hospitalization had no local alternative to the Negro Ward at City Hospital, which refused to allow African American physicians' practice privileges. The two nursing education programs in Winston-Salem, one at Baptist Hospital, the other at City Hospital, refused to admit African American students. In 1930, there were approximately 36,000 African Americans in Forsyth County and only 60 beds designated for African American patients in City Hospital, resulting in a patient-to-bed ratio of 600 to 1. In the 1930s, the situation was dire for African American patients and health care professionals.

Kate Bitting Reynolds Memorial Hospital (KBRMH)

"It was born in controversy, it lived in controversy, and it died in controversy," remarked Dr. Willard McCloud as he remembered the KBRMH (as cited in Luck, 2012, p. 1). To alleviate the crowded conditions in the African American wards at City Hospital, African

American community members wanted a new hospital staffed and managed by African American health professionals. The local white response was described in the May 1936 issue of *Southern Hospital*:

> Negro wards in Winston-Salem's City Memorial hospital have been badly crowded at times in recent months. Best solution of the problem appeared to be conversion of the present 180-bed unit into a Negro Hospital and construction of a 150-bed addition for white patients ... William Neal Reynolds ... gave $200,000, Richard Reynolds, Jr. ... promised $30,000 for a modern x-ray department. The Duke Endowment has appropriated $125,000 ["North Carolina," 1936, p. 48].

While the conversion of the old white section of the hospital into an African American hospital would help with overcrowding, the problem of African American patients being treated by white physicians who were not their primary care doctors remained. Demonstrating a forcefulness not seen in North Carolina up to this time, in 1936, officers of the Twin City Medical Society (TCMS), the local African American physicians' organization, met with Mayor W. T. Wilson to demand that African American physicians be allowed to treat their patients in the city-owned hospital. In addition, Dr. H. T. (Hobart Theodor) Allen, Dr. E. Shepherd Wright, and other officers of the TCMS spearheaded numerous petition drives to garner support for construction of a new African American hospital instead of inheriting an old building while a new hospital would be erected for white citizens. Fourteen physicians, six dentists, and four pharmacists—almost the entire membership of the TCMS—signed the organizations petition. Mrs. James Ellington led a citizen's petition drive to obtain the signatures of 100 leading local residents to request a new African American hospital rather than accept the old white hospital managed by white hospital administrators from City Hospital. Finally, nurses of the Edith Cavell Nursing Club, the local chapter of the National Association of Colored Graduate Nurses, under the leadership of nurses Morehead and Dillard, created their own petition in support of a new hospital (Grimes, 1972). These petitions along with a physician sit-in on the steps of City Hall convinced the Hospital Commission and the Board of Alderman to allow William Neal Reynolds, R.J. Reynolds' brother and President of Reynolds Tobacco Company, along with officers of the Duke Endowment, to fund the construction of a new city-owned African American hospital (Luck, 2012).

When the Kate Bitting Reynolds Memorial Hospital (KBRMH)

opened it was managed by the city's all-white Hospital Commission. Dr. J.B. Whittington, the white superintendent of the hospital, did not think African American health professionals were capable of independent practice and needed white physicians' and nurses' oversight (Grimes, 1972). African American health professionals were frustrated working in assistant and staff positions under white supervisors (Grimes, 1972). In 1939, Dr. J.C. Jordan and Dr. H.D. Malloy presented a list of grievances to the Hospital Commission, pointing out continuing racist practices at the hospital and highlighted those committed by Superintendent Whittington. For instance, when Dr. Hubert Eaton was an intern at the hospital, he noticed all of the interns were African Americans, and only white doctors were in the more advanced residency positions. Eaton asked hospital administrator Whittington about this discrepancy and was told, "There can be no colored resident doctors until we have an adequate number of colored nurses at the hospital because the hospital cannot permit colored resident doctors to give orders to our white nurses" (as cited in Ward, 2003, p. 75). No changes occurred as the result of Drs. Jordan and Malloy's meeting with Mr. Whittington.

As soon as KBRMH opened in July 1938, patient demand exceeded the facilities' capacity to treat all who sought care. In May 1940, Mr. W.N. Reynolds donated an additional $75,000 for a 96-bed expansion. However, being sympathetic to the African American staff's frustrations, Reynold's donation came with conditions (Historic marker, 2016). He wrote to Mayor Fain and the Board of Aldermen that the purposes of the hospital must include:

> Affording Negro physicians an opportunity to improve their professional qualifications and to treat their own hospital cases in this institution ... whenever it is practical to do so, and competent Negro physicians are available for the service, this hospital shall be placed entirely under the direction of Negro physicians and their assistants and that likewise, when it is practical to do so, and a competent Negro nurse is available for the purpose, a Negro superintendent of nurses shall be selected [as cited in Grimes, 1972, p. 378].

While government officials accepted Mr. Reynolds donation, his desire for African American administrators was ignored. By 1943, several members of the African American community talked about staging a public protest against the hospital. In an effort to head off the protest, the Hospital Commission appointed a 15-man Negro Advisory Committee which promptly submitted a list of recommendations for improvements at KBRMH. Unfortunately, the Committee's recommendations were ignored. The committee resubmitted their recommendations several months later, again, without results.

On October 9, 1945, after presenting the Hospital Commission with list of grievances, KBRMH student nurses went on strike (Grimes, 1972). The strike was short lived. Fearing their dismissal from the program, the students apologized for their actions and withdrew their grievances. Writing and presenting their grievances, and then going on strike, reflected the depth of nursing student's frustration over racist hospital and school of nursing policies. The same day the nursing students went on strike, a group of African American citizens met with Mayor George Lentz to express their objections to the way KBRMH was being managed. These actions led to the Hospital Commission's meeting with the Negro Advisory Board the next day, October 10, 1945. Attorney Hosea Price protested the conditions at the hospital remarking: "The hospital is filthy, dirty, nasty and not conducive to health. I do not believe that the donors intended it to be run as it is" (as cited in Grimes, 1972, p. 379). Shortly after this meeting, the Hospital Commission voted to employ an African American hospital administrator beginning July 1, 1946 (Grimes, 1972). Finally, after almost a decade of determined protests, the African American staff and their white benefactors achieved their desired outcome of African American leadership at KBRMH.

The number and quality of services at the hospital increased at the hospital from the late 1940s though the late 1950s. KBRMH was a major clinical training site for many health occupations. The nursing school maintained an "A" rating from the North Carolina Board of Nursing and over 100 young female graduates of the KBRMH School of Nursing earned the title Registered Nurse. The American Hospital Association and its Council on Medical Education accredited KBRMH and its three-year surgical residency program. In addition, the American Registry of Radiologic Technologists accredited the hospital's two-year program in x-ray technology (Grimes, 1972).

Overcrowding and aging facilities became major issues at both the African American KBRMH and the white City Memorial Hospital (originally opened in 1914 with a major addition in 1921) by the late 1950s (Prichard, 2016). Statistics taken from the KBRMH's annual reports show a quadrupling of adult in-patients and a ten-fold increase in emergency room visits between 1939 and 1963.

Annual Reports of the Kate B. Reynolds Memorial Hospital, 1940 and 1964

	1939	1963
Adult in-patients	2,768	8,676
Minor operations	862	1,855
Major operations	506	766
Emergency Room visits	1,967	19,570

In 1959, the R.J. Reynolds Tobacco Company donated land to the city of Winston-Salem for a new hospital on South Hawthorne Road, an area populated almost exclusively by whites. As Rauhauser-Smith (2012) noted: "The plan called for the purchase of 77 acres along Silas Creek Parkway, well out of downtown, a fact not lost on many including local newspapers who decried the move as racially motivated" (p. 1). City officials planned to construct a new hospital for white citizens and convert the old City Memorial Hospital to an African American hospital to replace KBRMH (Grimes, 1972). The majority of voters approved this plan, however, it was met with strong resistance from many in the African American community and their white allies. In 1963, as the new hospital was being constructed, the city's Board of Aldermen accepted a proposal from the Hospital Commission to erect a new $6 million dollar African American KBRMH rather than renovate the old City Memorial Hospital for the city's African American residents. City Memorial Hospital closed in May 1964 when the new Forsythe Memorial Hospital opened (Prichard, 2016).

Although the Civil Rights Act of 1964 and the Medicare and Medicaid programs enacted in 1965 forbade segregation in municipally owned hospital facilities, the city continued building the new Reynolds Memorial Hospital on Highland Avenue in a largely African American residential section of town. The new 250-bed, $6 million hospital was dedicated on January 16, 1970, and opened for patients on January 29, 1970. It primarily served the African American community. Reynolds Hospital was fully accredited by all of the major state and national accrediting organizations (Grimes, 1972, Prichard, 2016). However, there were too few patients and not enough income to support two (primarily racially) separate county-owned, publicly funded hospitals in Winston-Salem in the late 1960s and early 1970s. On October 2, 1971, ownership of Reynolds Hospital was transferred from the Forsythe County Hospital Authority to Forsyth County, and the facility was soon used for out-patient family health services and long term care instead of as a general hospital. In 1972, Forsythe Memorial Hospital became the only municipally owned hospital in Winston-Salem and served all citizens regardless of race (City of Winston-Salem, 2016).

Wilson, Wilson County

The earliest known residents of the land that is now known as Wilson County were the Tuscarora. With the settlement of Europeans on their ancestral lands, members of the Tuscarora Tribe suffered many hardships, including loss of hunting and fishing lands, disease, kidnappings, rape, beatings, murder, and Native slavery. The Tuscarora, fighting with several other tribes against the Europeans, engaged in the Tuscarora Wars of 1711–1713. The Native Americans were defeated and most moved out of the area, reducing their number from an estimated 6,000 to only several hundred (History, 2013). Large swaths of fertile land were open for Europeans and African slaves to cultivate.

In 1860, at the eve of the Civil War, Wilson County was home to 7,718 people; almost half were African American. There were 280 free African Americans and 3,494 enslaved people (Ptak, 2010). This racial division would remain stable for decades. Cigarettes, a recently invented tobacco product, were included in Civil War rations for both Union and Confederate troops. Soldiers from around the country developed a taste for Bright leaf tobacco, grown and cured primarily in eastern North Carolina, and the national demand for Bright leaf cigarettes exploded in the decades around the turn of the 20th century. The population of Wilson, a coastal plains town about forty miles east of Raleigh, grew from approximately 2,000 people in 1880 to 10,000 by 1910 with tobacco-related activities providing most of the employment gains in the county. Around 1900, Wilson became known as the "world's greatest tobacco market" (Lewis, 2013, p. 1).

Tobacco was a labor intensive crop before the mechanization that occurred after World War II. As the size and number of tobacco farms increased, the number of African American, low-wage, farm laborers also increased. The 1910 census shows an almost equal racial makeup of the county with 15,902 white residents and 13,350 African American citizens, one of few things that was racially equal in Wilson County from Reconstruction until the Civil Rights era. Wilson Sanitarium, the town's first hospital, opened in 1896 and refused to admit African

Americans. The only hospital in the state accepting African American patients in 1896 was St. Agnes Hospital in Raleigh, a 40-mile wagon trip over rough and unpaved roads (McKinney, 2010).

The town of Wilson was home to four incarnations of an African American hospital on East Green Street between 1905 and 1964. Founded because African Americans were banned from the existing white-only Wilson Sanitarium, the hospitals for African Americans chronically suffered from financial hardship in the days before the federal government and private insurance companies paid most hospital bills. Dr. Hargrave's Hospital began as an African American, physician-owned institution. However, by the 1930s, white physicians had taken ownership, renamed it Mercy Hospital and maintained the hospital so there would be no need to have a Negro wing of the white hospital in town (Valentine, 2002). Only after the *Simkins v. Moses Cone* court case and the enactment of the Civil Rights Act of 1964 were all citizens of Wilson County given the opportunity for similar treatment in a facility of their choice.

Dr. Hargrave's Hospital, 1905–1913

Fortunately for the African American people in and around Wilson, in 1903, Dr. Frank Settle Hargrave moved to town. Dr. Hargrave was born on August 27, 1874, in Lexington, North Carolina, and graduated from Leonard Medical School in 1901. His specialties were obstetrics and surgery. After practicing two years in Winston-Salem at Slater Hospital, Dr. Hargrave moved to Wilson and opened an office (Beckford, 2011). In May 1905, he bought a 16-room house on East Green Street and renovated the building for use as a clinic and hospital. In addition to practicing medicine in an underserved area of eastern North Carolina, Dr. Hargrave was very active in professional organizations on the state and national levels (Bailey, 1983). Dr. Hargraves was elected president of the Old North State Medical Society in 1912 and of the National Medical Association in 1914 (Beckford, 2011).

Wilson Hospital and Tubercular Home, 1913–Mid–1920s

Dr. Hargrave quickly realized that his private hospital could not adequately meet the need for hospitalization for the region's African

American population. He spearheaded a drive to build a new, larger, and more modern hospital. In 1913, Dr. Hargrave conveyed his building to the Trustees of the new Wilson Hospital and Tubercular Home (WHTH). The Trustees included Dr. Hargrave and two local businessmen, Mr. S.H. Vick and Mr. J.D. Reid. The old wooden structure was demolished and replaced by a two-story brick building with sunporches on each level. The Trustees took out a mortgage to help cover the $1,400 cost of construction, as well as money needed to purchase supplies and equipment and fund the hospital staff payroll.

An article from the *Wilson Times*, reprinted in the October 7, 1914, *Fayetteville Weekly Observer* provided details about opening day at the new hospital:

> On Tuesday about 500 visitors of both races passed through the new hospital just opened, and reception room to wards, and from wards to operating room, thence to kitchen and dining room they expressed themselves as being perfectly satisfied that they had inspected a hospital which in appointments and general fitness easily ranks with the best of such institutions in the state. The simple beauty and brightness had the effect upon the people of making them merry, and it was with difficulty that their mirth and hilarity were suppressed, which was made necessary by the condition of a patient who had just undergone an operation on opening day ["Wilson Hospital Formally Opened," 1914, p. 3].

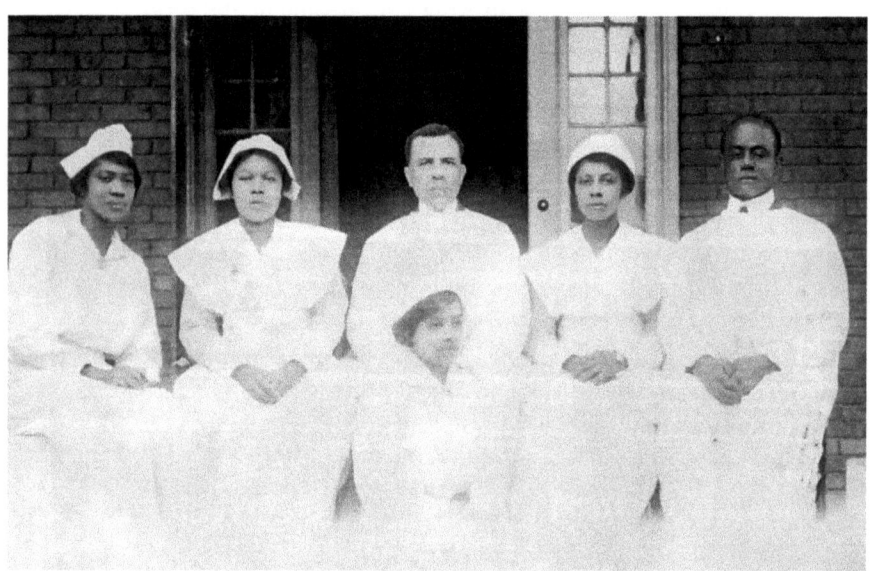

Staff of Wilson Hospital, Wilson, ca. 1930 (courtesy Oliver Nestus Freeman Round House Museum, Wilson, North Carolina).

The institution also garnered national attention. An item in the January 1914 *Journal of Outdoor Life: The Anti-Tuberculosis Magazine*, titled "Colored tuberculosis hospital open," read:

> After more than two years of incessant labor, a little group of colored men and women in Wilson, North Carolina, headed by Dr. F.S. Hargrave and Prof. Reid saw the realization of their dreams on September 22nd in the opening and dedication of the administrative building of the Wilson Hospital and Tubercular Home. This is the first and only private hospital for tuberculosis negroes in the United States. The funds for its erection and maintenance were collected entirely by the colored people themselves, a fact which is also unique. The hospital will have accommodations for about 20 patients and will be expanded from time to time as funds will permit [Colored tuberculosis, 1914, p. 349].

There were 10-bed wards for men, women and children as well as 15 private rooms. The building was described as an 80-foot wide, 90-foot deep, two-story, red brick building with upper and lower porches and massive white columns. One author concluded the new hospital was a "magnificent structure of beauty and strength" ("Wilson Hospital Formally Opened," 1914, p. 3).

In January 1915, the Wilson Board of Aldermen voted to appropriate $25 a month for the hospital, noting the hospital was doing a "splendid work" for the African Americans in the county ("Aid for Negro hospital," 1915, p. 5). Dr. W.A. Mitchner joined Dr. Hargrave on the medical staff. In 1927, Dr. J.F. Cowan and his wife Annie Mae Cowan, RN, began working at the new facility. Other nurses who worked at the WHTH were St. Agnes Hospital School of Nursing graduates Dinah Ada Adams and Henrietta Colvert, RN (Lewis, 1998).

Few if any patients in the WHTH had insurance or enough money to pay their bills in full. The hospital had to pay staff, buy supplies and equipment, feed the patients, and keep the building and grounds in working order. Money was a constant problem. By 1924, the hospital, being unable to pay its mortgage debts, went into foreclosure. Dr. Hargrave bought the building in a foreclosure auction for $7,000 using a loan from the town's only African American bank. When the bank failed in the late 1920s due to the nationwide financial hardships of the Great Depression, Dr. Hargrave again lost the hospital and soon moved to New Jersey in 1924. Dr. Hargrave practiced medicine and served in the New Jersey state legislature on and off from 1929 until he died in office in 1942 at age 60 ("A place," 1996).

Wilson Colored Hospital, 1927–1929

In 1927, Oliver Nestus Freeman, a local African American stone and brick mason of great renown, bought the hospital building and reopened it as the Wilson Colored Hospital. Unfortunately, the same financial issues that plagued Dr. Hargrave and his colleagues contributed to the closure of the Wilson Colored Hospital in 1929 (Lewis, 1998).

Mercy Hospital, 1930–1964

The fourth incarnation of the hospital for African Americans in Wilson began in 1930 when a group of local white citizens, including Dr. C.A. Woodard, Dr. L.V. Grady, Mr. William Clark, Mr. R.P. Watson, and one African American, Mr. William Hines, bought the building and reopened it as Mercy Hospital. Mr. Hines became the hospital's administrator in 1930 and stayed through the hospital's closure in 1964. Debts were paid off by private contributors, and for the first time, the town and county of Wilson both committed funds to support the hospital. In addition, the Duke Endowment gave the new Mercy Hospital one dollar a day for each charity patient, thus covering about a third of the costs of running the hospital (Valentine, 2002).

In 1938, the Trustees of Mercy sold the hospital to the town of Wilson in order to be eligible for a $16,000 grant from the federal government, the foundation of a $27,000 improvement campaign. The new money was partially used to increase the bed capacity from 25 to 40. The hospital had several wards, and there were no private rooms. The wards were surgery, a male ward, a female ward, a five-bed maternity ward, the nursery and pediatrics. St. Agnes Hospital School of Nursing graduate Mrs. Roxanna Exum, R.N., was hired as the Director of Nursing in 1943 and stayed through the hospital's closure in 1964. Mrs. Exum recalled that in 1943 the staff worked 12-hour shifts six days a week and got a half day off on the seventh day. They also got one weekend off each month ("A place," 1996). Although the facilities had improved and African Americans nurses worked in the hospital, at least one recorded racial atrocity occurred in 1949.

Mr. Fred Davis, Jr., a college-educated, World War II veteran, and an activist in voter registration drives for African Americans in Wilson County, was hit by a car on February 7, 1949, while he was riding a bicycle. McKinney (2010, p. 53) gives this account of the ensuing events.

> His family rushed him the East Wilson's Mercy Hospital and contacted a white doctor to come examine him. Davis—who sustained severe injuries—waited in vain for hours before Dr. Butterfield contacted a second, African American, doctor. Upon learning of the first phone call to the white doctor, the black doctor refused to come to the hospital and assist his friend and fraternity brother, citing a concern that the white doctor might be offended by his presence. Finally, after waiting nearly half a day, the white doctor arrived to examine Davis, performed a cursory exam and left. Davis died a short time later of massive internal bleeding. Looking back on that day in 1949, we cannot be certain of the motives carried by each doctor. Nor can we be certain of the fact that Davis's political activity played a factor in his death. However, one thing is quite clear, a system of racial custom and deference was capable of producing terror by both acts of commission and omission [p. 53].

Where overt racist attitudes were found, care suffered and outcomes were poorer than in hospitals with a record of interracial cooperation and harmony. While increasing the bed capacity and improving the quality of supplies and equipment, African American hospitals were improving the materiality of African American healthcare, perhaps the most important factor was interacting and at times challenging the attitudes of white physicians, nurses, and hospital administrators. The statistics below reflect the importance of adequate funding, and perhaps, racial attitudes—since the physicians working in Mercy Hospital also practiced in one of the other two white hospitals—had on patient outcomes in the 1940s.

Selected Results of the *Hospital Survey of Wilson County,* 1945

	Mercy Hospital (African American)	*Carolina General Hospital (White)*	*Woodard Hospital (White)*
Death rate	10.5	2.5	2.0
Average cost of treatment per patient	$2.88	$7.17	$7.80

The next major improvement at Mercy Hospital occurred in 1956. The Town of Wilson sold the hospital back to the Trustees, so they could apply for a $19,000 grant from the Ford Foundation. That money paid for an additional 10 beds for the hospital. In the 1950s, the number of employees hovered around eight (Baily, 1983). Mr. Hines was the administrator and he had a secretary, Mrs. Connie Freeman Banks.

Mrs. Roxanna E. Exum, R.N. was the Director of Nursing, Celeste McClain, R.N. Helen James, RN, Bessie Whitted, R.N., Frances Green, R.N., and Helen Wilson, R.N. were some of the nurses who worked at Mercy Hospital. There was not a permanent medical staff, but area white and African American physicians used the operating room and delivery suite for their patients. Local African American physicians who used Mercy Hospital included Dr. B.O. Barnes, Dr. Sullivan, Dr. Mitchner, and Dr. Cowan ("A place," 1996).

The 1963 *Simkins v. Moses Cone* court decision held that hospitals receiving public funds, such as Hill-Burton monies and later Medicaid and Medicare dollars, could not segregate patients or deny employment based on race. The decision of the court case was reaffirmed by the enactment of the 1964 Civil Rights Act. Wilson County government officials opened the new Wilson Memorial Hospital in 1964. Initially, all African American patients and staff were assigned to the 3rd floor, but as that practice violated the law, it was changed within a year or so ("A place," 1996).

Today, the Wilson Hospital and Tubercular Home/Mercy Hospital building stands empty and is falling into disrepair. The building does not convey the drive, ingenuity, professionalism, and determination that Dr. Hargrave and the other physicians, nurses, and staff devoted to establishing and maintaining a place of healing for people shunned by those with power and money. The people helped and lives saved are the true legacy of Wilson Hospital and Tubercular Home (Carr, 2009).

Asheville, Buncombe County

Buncombe County is nestled in the middle of the Appalachian Mountains in North Carolina. It is home to Asheville, the largest city in the mountain region of the state. Despite the popular misconception that Appalachia has all white residents, the Appalachian, African American residents of Asheville have a long and proud history. During the Jim Crow era, African American hospitals and a school of nursing were part of the social fabric of Ashville (Pollitt & Leonard, 2014). The town of Asheville was founded after the Buncombe toll road was built in the late 1820s. According to the U.S. census of 1860, Buncombe County had 1,933 enslaved people and 111 free blacks for a total African

American population of 2,044 constituting 16.2 percent of Buncombe County's population at the eve of the Civil War (Waters, 2012). With the arrival of the railroad to Asheville Junction in 1880, Asheville transitioned from a rural outpost of approximately 2,000 settlers, who had wrested the land from the Cherokee less than a hundred years before, to a growing center of commerce and industry (Pollitt & Leonard, 2014).

Tuberculosis had become a serious national health crisis in the decades after the Civil War. The high altitude and thin mountains air were thought to help heal tubercular lungs. Asheville, like the sand hills region in southeastern North Carolina, became a health destination with many tuberculosis sanatoria (Pollitt & Leonard, 2014). By 1930, Asheville was home to 14,260 African Americans who made up about 28 percent of the city's total population (Waters, 2012).

Torrence Hospital, 1910–1915

The short-lived and little known Torrence Hospital, first opened at 16 Eagle Street and moved to 95 Hill Street in 1911, was owned and operated by African American physician Dr. William Green Torrence (Davis & Ready, 1980). Dr. Torrence graduated from Shaw Institute in Raleigh, North Carolina and the Dearborn Medical College in Chicago. He arrived in Asheville in 1907, opened an office in the Young Men's Institute Building, and started a practice. Dr. Torrence opened his hospital in 1910 ("Funeral of Dr. Torrence," 1915). He lived with his family on the first floor and had several rooms upstairs to board patients who needed his close attention (Davis, 1980). Unfortunately, the Torrence Hospital closed in 1915 with Dr. Torrence's untimely death from tuberculosis at age 34 ("Colored physician," 1915).

Circle Terrace Sanatorium, 1912–1917

Dr. John Wakefield Walker, a 1902 Leonard Medical School graduate, established the first African American health care facility in Asheville to treat patients with tuberculosis. The Circle Terrace Sanatorium opened in 1912 (Pozner, 2015). A classified advertisement in the 1916 Asheville telephone directory described the facility:

> This is believed to be the only institution in the world for the exclusive treatment and care of tuberculosis for COLORED PEOPLE. Situated in the most

Part II—The Health Care Facilities

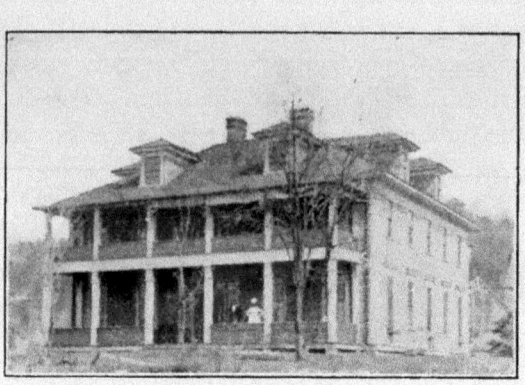

Circle Terrace Sanatorium

ASHEVILLE.. N. C.

J. W. Walker, M. D.
Physician in Charge

W. G. Torrence, M. D.
Consultant

THIS is believed to be the only institution in the world for the exclusive treatment and care of tuberculosis for COLORED PEOPLE.

Situated in the most perfect all-the-year-round climate that can be found for the treatment of tuberculosis.

The Sanatorium is conducted under the strict sanitary laws of the City of Asheville.

Electric lights, call bells, telephone, baths and other modern improvements.

Ample porches with south-eastern and south-western exposure.

Moderate rates. Mrs. Carrie Robinson, an experienced nurse, manager. For further information apply to J. W. WALKER, M. D.

Advertisement for Circle Terrace Sanatorium (Asheville City Directory, 1916).

perfect all-the-year-round climate that can be found for the treatment of tuberculosis. The Sanitarium is conducted under the strict sanitary laws of the City of Asheville. Electric lights, call bells, telephone, baths and other modern improvements. Ample porches with southeastern and southwestern exposure. Moderate rates. Mrs. Carrie Robinson, an experienced nurse, manager. For further information, apply to J.W. Walker, M.D. [p. 497].

Circle Terrace Sanatorium was closed by 1917. A fire destroyed the local African American school and the Sanatorium was used for temporary classrooms until a new school was opened ("Students," 2015). Dr. Walker accepted a position at the new Negro Division of the State Tuberculosis Sanitarium in Hoke County, NC. He stayed there three years before returning to Asheville. Upon his return, Dr. Walker opened a private practice but did not reopen his sanitarium (Mitchell, 2014).

Blue Ridge Hospital and School of Nursing, 1922–1928

The closing of Torrence Hospital in 1915, and the Circle Terrace Sanatorium in 1917, meant African Americans in Buncombe County were again without a hospital where their doctors of choice could treat them. A group of African American citizens in Buncombe County established the Blue Ridge Hospital and School of Nursing in 1922. The hospital began without any backing from white philanthropists or organizations. Nursing Superintendent Ruby Woodbury (n.d.) explained the hospital's primary objectives:

> The hospitalization of Negroes seeking surgical or medical treatment under the care and skill of their own doctors, to provide an opportunity for colored physicians to improve their technique and skill in keeping with the best medical and surgical thought of the day, to provide an opportunity for the efficient training of nurses and to serve as a nucleus for the promotion and dissemination of knowledge pertaining to hygiene and sanitation [p. 1].

No official papers have been found related to the school of nursing documenting its policies, curriculum or teaching staff. A single photograph identifies Flossie Metz, Lula Long, and Kathleen Wills as the first three graduates of the nursing program in 1925. North Carolina Board of Nursing records list Geneva Sitrena Collins (1930), Lois Rice Cunningham (1929), and Maude Beulah Du Pont (1926) as three other graduates of Blue Ridge Hospital's nursing program (First graduates, 1925).

Superintendent of Nursing Woodbury promoted Blue Ridge Hospital. In a pamphlet about the hospital, she wrote:

> The hospital is prepared to care for all the colored work in the city and county. The Mission Hospital is the only white institution in the city having colored wards. To be consistent in our aims and institutional life, we feel that the Blue Ridge Hospital is the logical place for all Negroes needing hospital treatment in the city and county. As a rule, the colored nurse is better qualified by nature to minister to her own race; with her there can be no thought of prejudice [Woodbury, n.d., p. 2].

The opening of Blue Ridge Hospital and School of Nursing demonstrated the dedication of Asheville's African American citizens to improve their community. An article in the *Asheville Citizen* reported that the new hospital cost $30,000 and opened with an indebtedness of $16,000. With its combination of private rooms, wards, and sun porches, the hospital was well-equipped to accommodate and as many as 30 patients ("Formal opening," 1922). The hospital had an operating room and dietary kitchen. Six African American physicians: Doctors White, Louis N. Gallego, Iee Otis Miller, John Walker Holt, a 1917 graduate of Leonard Medical School, Thompson, John Wakefield Walker, a 1902 graduate of Leonard Medical School, and Ruben H. Bryant, an 1889 graduate of Leonard Medical School, constituted the medical staff. Dr. Bryant served as Chief of Staff (Rives, 1922). The hospital opened in 1922 with Nurse Sadie Woods as its first Superintendent. Later Nursing Superintendents included Jeanette May (1924–25), Lula Long (1926), Mattie Sears (1927), Ruby Woodbury (1928), and Flossie Metz (1929–1930). Nurse Idell Tate was the night superintendent (*Asheville City Directories*, 1922–1930).

Hospital authorities asked the public to donate bed linens, food, and other helpful items ("Colored Hospital formally opened," 1922). Local women founded both the "The Hospital Guild" and the "Loyal Blue Club" to assist the hospital and its patients. Superintendent Woodbury (n.d.) wrote about the clubs in a brochure about the hospital:

> These clubs are composed of women whose services have been unsparing, and whose attention has been painstaking in rendering whatever aid is possible in caring for its [the hospital's] needs [Woodbury, n.d., p. 2].

In its first five years, 1,801 patients were treated at Blue Ridge Hospital. There were 854 surgical cases, 130 obstetrical cases, and 817 medical cases. The mortality rate was a very low 5 percent. The hospital charged patients for services, but no one was turned away due to lack of funds (Woodbury, n.d.). The statistics clearly indicate that the need for the hospital was great.

Despite the value and use of the Blue Ridge Hospital, it did not receive needed support from municipal funds. Both the Asheville City and Buncombe County governments allocated one dollar a day for charity care for impoverished residents needing hospitalization. Unfortunately, despite repeated requests from the administrators of Blue Ridge Hospital to be designated as the official charity hospital for African American citizens and, therefore, receive the fees the city and county government paid for indigent patients, both governmental bodies refused this request. Instead, they reimbursed only Mission Hospital for charity care (Marlowe, 2004). Blue Ridge Hospital could not raise enough money to both repay its debt and subsidize care for many of its patients. In 1928 it closed its doors. Dr. L.O. Miller, a physician at Blue Ridge at the time of its closing, laid significant blame at the feet of local government officials. He stated: "Our failure to interest the city and county officials to give us indigent patients, and the apparent lack of interest of Negro leaders in the hospital, forced us to close the institution" ("Close doors of Negro Hospital," 1930, p. 68). Clearly, there were complex political and racial dynamics at play. After Blue Ridge Hospital closed, the only hospital care available to African American Buncombe County residents was delivered in the segregated basement Negro Ward in Mission Hospital.

The Shuford Clinic

Dr. Mary Francis Polly Shuford was the only white, female, physician in North Carolina to establish a private hospital for African Americans. Dr. Shuford, from a prominent Asheville family, began advocating for a hospital for African Americans soon after she graduated from medical school in 1935. Some fellow physicians and family members discouraged Dr. Shuford's efforts even though there was a great need. An article in the *Asheville Citizen* illustrated the dismal state of hospitalization for local African Americans:

> Many times physicians with Negro patients have to wait for months to get a hospital bed for a major operative case. Minor operative cases are hardly worth considering in this situation.... Medical facilities for Negroes generally are almost hopelessly inadequate.... Helpless Negroes died because hospitalization couldn't be had when they needed it ["Negro Health," 1941, p. 3].

In May of 1941, using a substantial donation from a wealthy white friend, Shuford bought a nine-bedroom house at 269 College Street, renovated it, and opened the Shuford Clinic for Negroes. The Shuford Clinic consisted of an operating room, nine patient beds, a bedroom for two nurses, a kitchen, an examination room and offices. Two hundred operations and almost 2,000 outpatient visits occurred during the Shuford Clinic's first year. Shuford invited local African American physicians to use the facility but for unexplained reasons, none did (Durham, 1994).

The Asheville Colored Hospital

The patient census at the Shuford Clinic demonstrated the great need for a larger and more comprehensive hospital for African Americans in western North Carolina. The Clinic could neither see all the people who needed care, nor meet all the needs of those patients they did see within its limited facility. Shuford enlisted the help of her friend and *Asheville Citizen Times* newspaper publisher Charles Webb in advocating for an African American hospital in Asheville. Webb energized the community through a series of newspaper articles, editorials, and coaxed his Rotary Club into making the creation of the Asheville Colored Hospital a primary Club goal (Shuford, 1975).

Webb, publisher of both the *Asheville Citizen* and the *Asheville Times*, wrote a blistering editorial that ran in a joint Sunday edition of the both newspapers (1939). It read:

> For years now the people of Asheville have been talking piously about the need for more adequate hospital facilities for Negroes. The net results of all this discussion is the simple but ugly fact that the situation today is just as appalling as it ever was. Here are the disgraceful conditions—Asheville has five hospitals with 341 beds exclusive of beds for babies. From four of the hospitals Negroes are excluded altogether although they constitute a full third of the cities' population. They are admitted to only one hospital which has allotted 18 beds for them. Expressed in rough figures this means that while there is one bed for every one hundred white residents, there is only one bed for every one thousand Negro residents. If the Negro were free from the ills and accidents that afflict the rest of the human race, there might be some plausible justification for such shocking favoritism. But unhappily neither disease nor death knows any color line or obeys any Jim Crow laws.... Who is to blame? Many persons, many organizations, many groups are to blame. In some ways the whole white race of Asheville is to blame for we have complacently accepted a condition which we could have bettered and which impeaches our right to be classed as a truly civilized community.... The white physicians are blameworthy because they have not emphasized to all of us the utter indecency of the hospital situation as it related to the colored race. Is it too much to ask the doctors to show leadership in such matters? The city and county governments are very properly subject to criticism for they have not acted themselves or inspired others to act. Local governments have very direct and inescapable responsibilities in ensuring adequate hospitalization of all of the people, including Negroes. The governing bodies of the various local hospitals are not without sin in this situation. They have failed to take a sufficiently broad view of their opportunities and responsibilities [p. 20].

Shortly after publishing the editorial, Webb was appointed Chairman of the new Rotary Negro Hospital Committee. The Committee determined that $12,000 would be needed to build and equip an Asheville Colored Hospital (ACH). They started a fundraising drive. Their efforts were successful and more than $25,000 was donated to the hospital cause (Action, n.d.). African American citizens raised almost $3,000. African American school children contributed pennies at school to the hospital fundraising campaign. An article in the January 21, 1943, *Asheville Citizen* noted:

> The extraordinary response from the Negro citizens in this town and county to the financial appeal for the Asheville Colored Hospital is decidedly the most gratifying development of this campaign. The Negroes have already raised $2,500 dollars. This money has come largely out of the pitifully meager resources of their own people ["Colored committee raises fund," 1943, pp. 1–2].

The Duke Endowment contributed $2,500, and pledged to donate $1 a day for each charity patient cared for in the hospital, a pledge they were unwilling to make to the Blue Ridge Hospital a decade earlier (New Colored Hospital to open next week, 1943).

In 1943, the Rotary Committee purchased a two-story brick building on the corner of Southside Street and Biltmore Avenue, the former home and clinic of Dr. Reuben Bryant, one of the earliest African American physicians in Asheville. After remodeling the building, it became the 35-bed Asheville Colored Hospital. An article in the *Asheville Citizen Times* commented on the significance of this development:

> It will be the first time in the history of modern Asheville that anything approaching adequate hospital facilities for Negroes have been available here. It has not been possible to set an exact date for the opening but it is hoped that the institution can hold open house on the afternoon of October 14. That date falls on a Thursday, the day most domestic help has the afternoon off.... The hospital will start operations with a nest egg of $7,000. ["Colored hospital," 1943, p. B-8].

Over 1,500 people attended the hospital's opening celebrations on October 23, 1943. Four patients were brought in from the Shuford Clinic that day, and 12 patients were admitted the next day. Reminiscent of the early days of the Blue Ridge Hospital 20 years earlier, local residents donated appliances, equipment, and supplies. These donations included a Kelvinator (refrigerator), 128 pieces of silverware, baby clothes, a scale, flowers, a desk, two tables, six chairs, and a wheelchair (1,500 persons, 1943).

Fees were $2.50 a day for room and board, $6 for a delivery fee, and $1 to $3 for laboratory work. There were six-bed wards: one for children, one for obstetrical patients, two for adult men, and two for adult women. In addition, there were two private rooms for patients, one of which was furnished by the City Federation of Colored Women's Club, and named in honor of Fannie Bryant, widow of a well-loved African American physician and prior owner of the home that became the Asheville Negro Hospital. The Asheville Colored Hospital also housed an operating room, sterilizing room, kitchen, staff dining room, and rooms for the Superintendent of Nursing and another for physicians needing overnight accommodations. The back hall was remodeled into an Emergency Room. Six indoor bathrooms were installed and all the windows were rescreened (A Rotary started hospitals for Negroes, 1944).

All seven African American physicians in the city served on the hospital staff, with Dr. John P. Holt, a second-generation Asheville African American physician serving as Chief of Staff. Several white physicians in the area performed operations on an as-needed basis ("New Colored Hospital to open next week," 1943).

The first nursing supervisor was Mrs. Edna Miller, RN, a graduate of the Uniontown, Pennsylvania, Hospital School of Nursing. She was a white nurse who had been employed for 14 years at the local St. Joseph's Tuberculosis Sanatorium and Biltmore Hospital. The Asheville Colored Hospital also employed two unnamed African American graduate nurses, six African American nursing assistants, and two African American cooks ("New Colored Hospital to open next week," 1943). The hospital and its staff served the African American community of western North

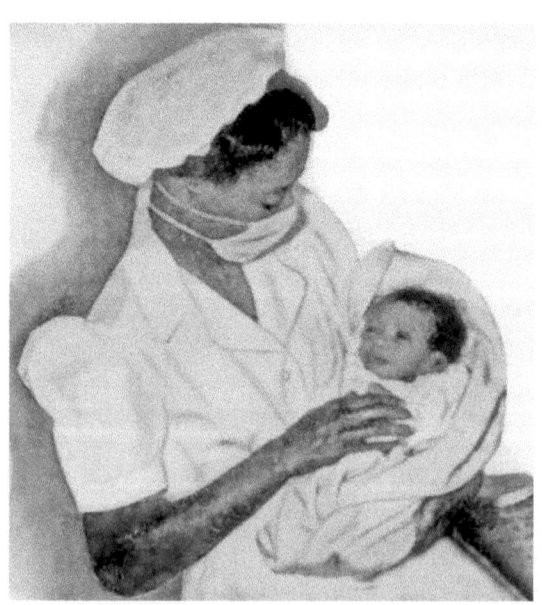

Nurse with newborn at Asheville Colored Hospital, ca. 1944 (*The Rotarian*, August 1944).

Carolina from its opening in October of 1943 until it merged with Mission Hospital and became the segregated Victoria Wing of Mission Memorial Hospital from 1951 through the mid–1960s. After 80 years, in the mid-1960s Mission Memorial Hospital began providing care and employment opportunities to all residents of western North Carolina regardless of race.

Henderson, Vance County

The original inhabitants of northern central North Carolina, the Occaneechi Indians, were forced off their homelands by war and disease. The land that became Vance County was settled by Europeans and enslaved African Americans by the early 1700s. Although Vance County, named for North Carolina's Confederate Civil War governor, was not formed until 1881, the counties that contributed land for the new county—Franklin, Granville, and Warren—had antebellum populations that were roughly evenly divided between whites and African Americans. At the turn of the 20th century, Vance County was rural, dotted with small towns, including Henderson, Dabney, and Kittrell (Blackburn, 1984).

Although the county built and maintained public schools for its white children after the Civil War, no schools for African American children existed until the Freedmen's Mission Board of the United Presbyterian Church opened the Henderson Industrial Institute in 1891 (Campbell, 1995). The school remained the only high school African Americans could attend in Vance County until 1970. Vance County African Americans also faced exclusionary policies in local hospitals. Both the Sarah Elizabeth Hospital, founded in 1912, and the Maria Parham Hospital, established in 1926, refused to admit African Americans until the Civil Rights Act of 1964 was enforced in 1966. Once again, the United Presbyterian Church, this time under the guise of the Women's General Missionary Society (WGMS), stepped up to provide basic human services for African Americans in Vance County by opening and supporting Jubilee Hospital from 1911 until 1966 (Ragland, 1991).

Jubilee Hospital, 1911–1966

In 1910, a tragic and unnecessary death of a student with appendicitis at the Henderson Industrial Institute was the catalyst for the founding of Jubilee Hospital in Henderson, North Carolina. The closest hospital that would accept African American patients was Lincoln Hospital in Durham, NC, a 40-mile wagon trip over rutted and rocky roads. The student's physician thought the trip would be fatal, but it turned out the appendectomy he performed in the patient's home did not save her life (Peace, 1956). Believing that an operation in a hospital's sterile environment could have prevented a student's death, the principal of the institute, the Rev. John Adam Cotton, donated a plot of his own land for a hospital building and the WGMS of the United Presbyterian Church raised funds to build and equip the new hospital. Because most of the funds were raised in 1911, the 50th anniversary, or "Jubilee year," of the start of the Civil War, which brought freedom to people enslaved in the Southern states, the hospital was named Jubilee Hospital (JH) (Ragland, 1991). In the September 1911 issue of *The Women's Missionary Magazine*, Mrs. Samuel Yourd made this appeal for funds for Jubilee Hospital:

> The rooms, while not large will be light and airy. The whole building will be heated with hot air and lighted with electricity or gas. There is a bath room on each floor.... There will be needed in the way of furnishings—office furniture, a table and six chairs for the dining room ... nine ward beds ... four to six children's beds, instruments, an operating table, wheel chair ... [p. 39].

The fundraising campaign was successful. The new hospital had 15 beds, as well as an operating room, dining room, and kitchen. Dr. John Earl Baxter, a 1905 graduate of Leonard Medical School, was the first physician and Daisy Reed, RN, was the first Superintendent of Nursing. Nurse Reed was followed by Eva Johnson Adams, RN, in 1913 who directed nursing at JH for almost 50 years, retiring in 1961. Dr. Samuel McDonald Beckford, a surgeon, joined the staff in 1919. Although all patients were African Americans, local physicians of both races cared for patients at Jubilee. Other physicians on the staff included Paul S. Green, William E. Green, Jr., James P. Green, Rubert N. Venable, and Parnell N. Avery. An article in the March 1916 issue of the *Women's Missionary Magazine* reported that 316 patients had been treated at JH in 1915, an increase of 73 from the 243 people cared for in 1914. In 1915, surgeons performed 119 major and 83 minor operations and 21 women delivered their babies at the hospital. Only nine patients died that year ("Henderson, N.C.," 1916). The hospital was a general community hospital that treated medical, surgical, maternity, gynecological, orthopedic, and later tubercular patients.

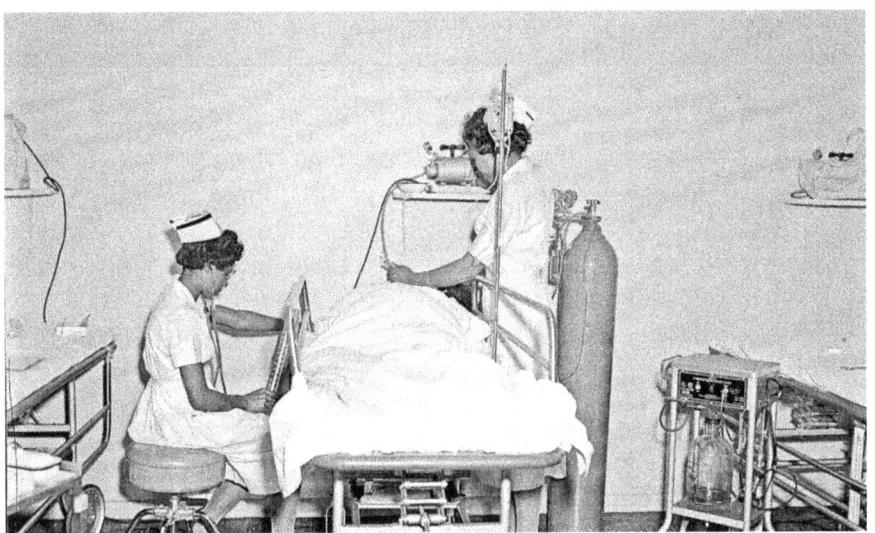

Nurses providing bedside care at Jubilee Hospital, Henderson, ca. 1950s. *Jubilee Hospital Welcomes You*, booklet, 1963. (United Presbyterian Church in the U.S.A. Support Agency, Division of Communications–Interpretation, Dept. of Mission Interpretation Records, 1939–1978, RG 303.1, box 2, folder 48, Presbyterian Historical Society, Philadelphia, PA).

Nurses training, a vital function of the hospital, began in 1918. Eva Johnson Adams, RN, Nursing Superintendent, described the situation in a 1921 article:

> ... we now have four girls in training. One has almost completed the three year course, and we are very proud of her and regret very much to see her leave, but are glad to have such as she goes out from our institution, knowing she will be a shining star. This training is quite necessary, not only to the nurses and their families, but to the communities they enter. A great many lives are lost each year through ignorance of care of the sick ["Henderson Hospital," 1921, p. 177].

Elizabeth Viola Davis, Hettie Jim Hunt, Ida Mae Plummer, and Carrie L. Alexander were some of Jubilee's graduates who earned the registered nurse credential. The school was closed in the 1930s, because standards for accreditation rose beyond the means of the hospital. Other registered nurses who worked at Jubilee included Maggie Esther Smith, Magnolia B. Barnett, Cleo Betsch, Matilda Lawrence, Mary Hargrave, Gertrude Allen, and Joan Hacker. Mary Carpenter, RN, a white nurse, became the Superintendent of Nurses in 1963 (Hughes, 1988).

In 1929, using funds donated from both the Duke Endowment and the Women's Mission Board of the United Presbyterian Church, a tuberculosis wing and later a maternity ward were added to the hospital. In the 1930s, a new operating room, x-ray equipment, and a laboratory provided additional services for local people (Hughes, 1988). The Reverend Cotton, justifiably proud of the institution he helped create, remarked, "Through Jubilee, wounds and bruises are bound up, the suffering are relieved, the sick healed and the poor and needy helped" (Jubilee Hospital, 1963, p. 2).

In addition to the hospital's mission of providing physical care for those in need, and nursing education for local women, spiritual care was a daily part of the hospital routine. Although JH was owned and supported by the United Presbyterian Church, patients of all races and faiths were welcome. The pastor of the local Cotton Memorial United Presbyterian Church also served as the hospital chaplain, but leaders of all faiths were welcomed to provide pastoral care for their hospitalized congregants within JH. Daily devotionals services were held in the hospital for any staff and patients who were able to attend. Later, when

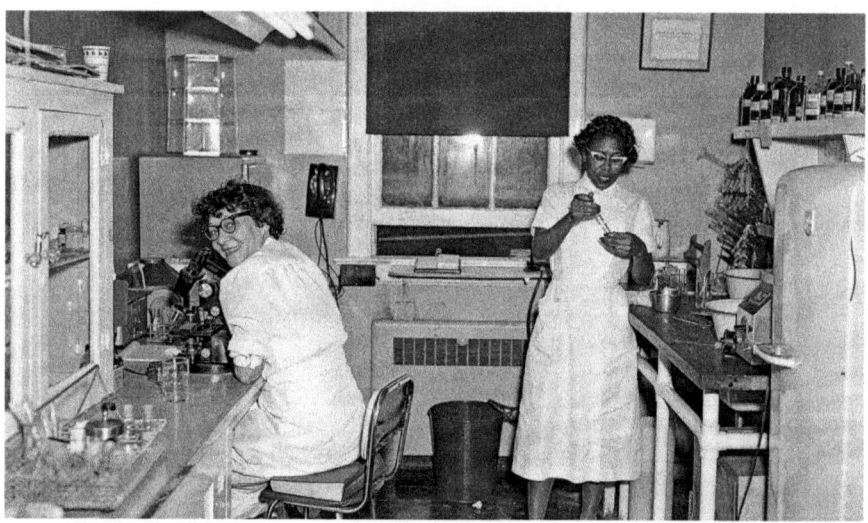

Laboratory technicians at Jubilee Hospital in Henderson, ca. 1950s. *Jubilee Hospital Welcomes You*, booklet, 1963 (United Presbyterian Church in the U.S.A. Support Agency, Division of Communications–Interpretation, Dept. of Mission Interpretation Records, 1939–1978, RG 303.1, box 2, folder 48, Presbyterian Historical Society, Philadelphia, PA).

an intercom was installed in the hospital, it was used to broadcast short daily services. The hospital chaplain was also available for visitation in patient rooms and passed out religious literature (House of healing, 1963).

Throughout the hospital's existence, the WGMS regularly published requests for supplies and equipment for Jubilee Hospital in their monthly journal. United Presbyterian women's groups and Sunday Schools classes responded enthusiastically to these requests. These groups sewed and donated clothing, layettes, linens, bandages and other useful items to JH ("Missionary society," 1947, "Golden rule class," 1963). In a 1926 article titled "Shower of linens and money," the following items were among those listed as donated to the hospital: 13 quilts, 184 Turkish towels, 87 diapers, and 17 dolls.

In 1950, in addition to the 16 physicians and two dentists who had privileges at Jubilee, the staff was comprised of a Director of Nursing, four registered nurses, three practical nurses, eight nurse's aides/orderlies, a laboratory technician, an X-ray technician, food service workers, a cleaning staff, and a hospital administrator with several secretaries ("House of Healing in North Carolina," 1963).

Few improvements were made to the facility during the Great Depression or World War II. By 1950, the building was condemned but was allowed to remain open until a replacement was completed in 1959. The new Jubilee Hospital, built with funds from the Duke Endowment, federal Hill-Burton Act monies, and local and church donations, boasted 30 beds, six bassinets, a laboratory, nursery, staff dining room, kitchen, office, lounges, and operating, recovery, delivery and emergency rooms (Hughes, 1988).

Mrs. Eva Adams, who served as Nursing Supervisor of Jubilee Hospital for over 30 years, shared some interesting stories from the hospital:

> About a month ago, a white physician in an adjoining county, brought an obstetrical case to us about midnight. It was a deformed humped-back girl who was wonderfully ignorant. She could neither read nor write, has no mother.... She could not be delivered normally and the surgeons had to make an abdominal delivery ... mother and baby are both getting along well at the hospital at this time. About two months ago, the welfare officer here, a very fine Christian white woman brought a white baby about a week old. She said a girl from a good family in another town had made a mistake [was pregnant and unmarried].... She asked us to keep the baby and not let any white person see it until she could find a home for it [Adams, 1960, p. 798].

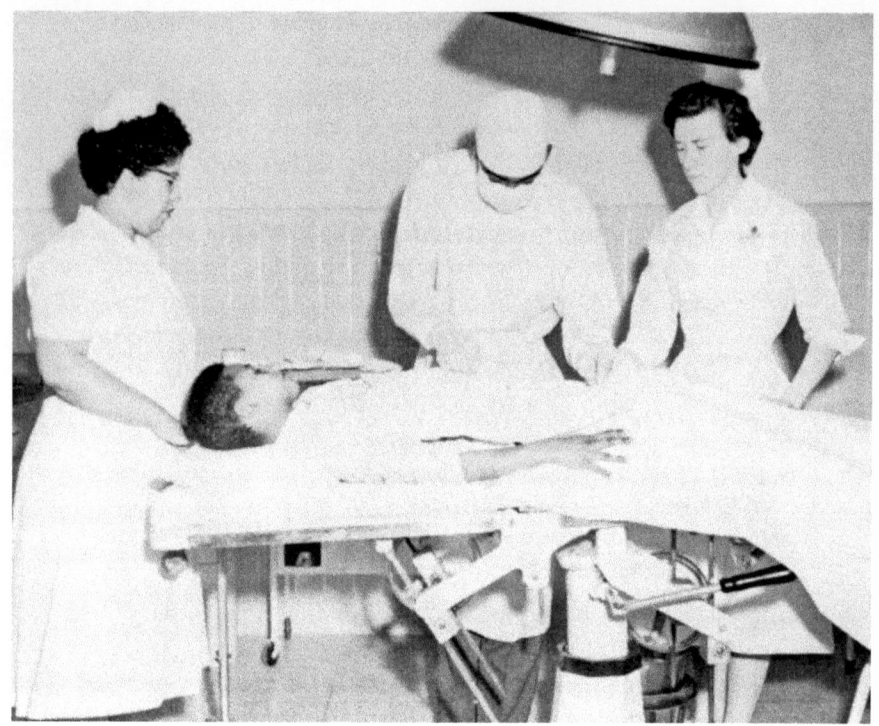

Physician and nurses performing an operation at Jubilee Hospital, Henderson, ca. 1960s. *Jubilee Hospital Welcomes You*, booklet, 1963 (United Presbyterian Church in the U.S.A. Support Agency, Division of Communications–Interpretation, Dept. of Mission Interpretation Records, 1939–1978, RG 303.1, box 2, folder 48, Presbyterian Historical Society, Philadelphia, PA).

A pamphlet titled "House of Healing in North Carolina" produced by the Presbyterian Church in 1963 reported:

> The long, low, lines of the red brick building present an attractive appearance, while inside the hospital an atmosphere of quiet efficiency and competence prevails ... equipped to treat ordinary short-term ailments, Jubilee can handle medical, surgical, gynecological, and orthopedic cases.... Most of the people Jubilee serves live in rural areas and work in low-income jobs as tenant farmers and laborers ... almost one third of the total number of patients treated at Jubilee last year were welfare patients [pp. 2–3].

Between October 1961 and September 1962, the hospital cared for 1,950 inpatients and 2,000 outpatients. In addition to caring for people needing hospitalization, hospital personnel sought to meet other needs of their clientele. Working with the Vance County Public

Health Department, the hospital hosted and housed several clinics including those for pre-natal care and tuberculosis screenings. In the summer of 1962, Mrs. Adams, the Superintendent of Nurses, conducted a six-week, 30-hour home nursing course open to all the women in the community. The pamphlet further reported on the Jubilee staff members' role in a voter registration campaign:

> Several members of Jubilee's administrative and medical staff are active in a county-wide voter's league which has been influential in promoting voter registration among Negroes in the area [p. 6].

These voter registration efforts demonstrate yet another positive impact African American hospitals and staff had on their communities.

The new hospital, costing over $425,000, was only used for seven years, until 1966, when Civil Rights legislation forced the white-only Maria Parham Hospital to accept people of all races for care. The beds from JH were sent to a Presbyterian missionary hospital in Egypt (Phillippe, 2015). The facility was empty for 15 years until it was renovated for use as a municipal building in 1981.

Monroe, Union County

Quality Hill Sanatorium, 1912–1941

After the Waxhaw and Catawba Native American tribes had been decimated by smallpox and war, the land comprising Union County was settled by German, Scotch-Irish, English, and Welch pioneers along with enslaved peoples. Union County was formed in 1842 and in the 19th and early 20th centuries, was rural with several small towns, including Monroe, Fairview and Wingate (Walden, 1964). At the beginning of the Civil War, Union County had a total population of 11,202. Of those, 2,246 were enslaved and 53 were free African Americans, comprising about 20 percent of the total population. By the turn of the 20th century, Union County had approximately 27,000 residents of which about 12,000 were African Americans ("Union County History," 2015).

Monroe, the county seat, was the only town with hospitals. In 1903, white Drs. John Monroe, J.E. Ashcraft, and H.D. Stewart opened the 16-room Stewart-Ashcraft Sanitarium on the second floor of a downtown building, but it closed by 1907 (American Medical, 1909; Union County Medical, 1968). Surprisingly, the first substantial hospital to operate in Union County was the African American Quality Hill Sanatorium (QHS), owned by Dr. John Sherman Massey. He was born in neighboring Lancaster County, South Carolina, on May 30, 1866, to Tom and Mary Massey, newly freed slaves. Dr. Massey moved to Monroe shortly after graduating from Leonard Medical School in 1896 and began seeing patients in their homes ("Dr. John Sherman Massey," 2016). At that time, the closest hospitals for both races were in Charlotte, a 25-mile wagon ride away. Uniquely, it appears that Dr. Massey was a member of the Union County Medical Society (UCMS). He is the only recorded North Carolinian, African American physician in the Jim Crow era who was a member of an otherwise all-white county medical society. The October 1903 minutes of the UCMS note that Dr. Massey was not in attendance and the June 1912 minutes show he led the group's monthly discussion ("John S. Massey, M.D.," 2012).

The first public mention of QHS was in the March 26, 1912, edition of the local newspaper, *The Monroe Journal.* The paper published a letter to the editor under the title, "Dr. Massey asks for aid":

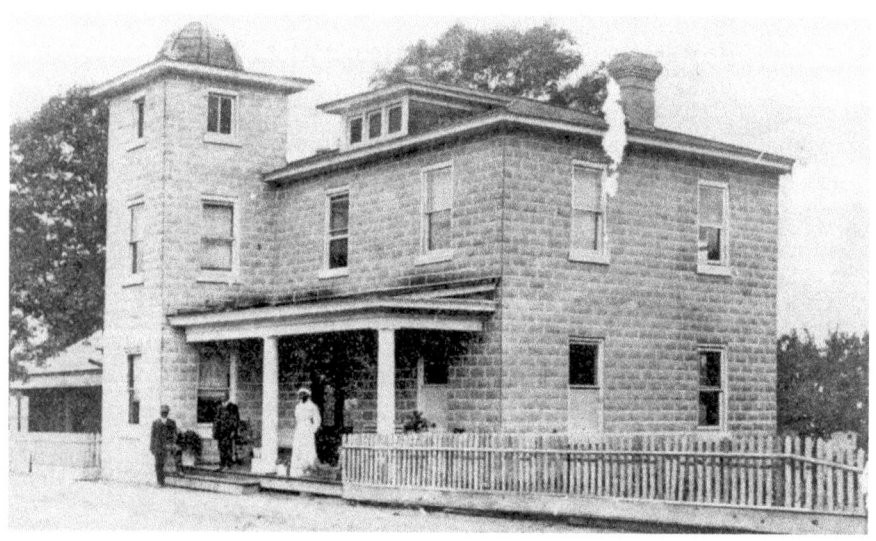

Quality Hill Sanatorium, Monroe, North Carolina, ca. 1912 (courtesy State Archives of North Carolina).

To my white friends of Monroe and union county: I wish to state that I am erecting a small sanitarium in the city of Monroe, N.C. containing ten rooms, and two stories. One or two of these will be devoted to charity, therefore I appeal to the generous, open hearted and benevolent white friends of Monroe and the county for a donation. Any amount given will be received and highly appreciated. Thanking you in advance for any favors shown. I remain Yours Respectfully, Dr. J.S. Massey [Massey, 1912, p. 1].

The building progressed quickly. In the July 23, 1912, issue of *The Monroe Journal*, a notice announced that QHS would "open its doors to the public for inspection on Monday August 19th" ("Opening of Sanitarium," 1912, p. 1). In that same notice, Dr. Massey asked for donations of money, linens, and crockery. A week later, July 30, 1912, an item in *The Charlotte Observer* described the building as "concrete and quite commodious" ("A colored hospital," p. 10).

The Journal of the National Medical Association mentioned QHS in the Society and Personal column in its October-December 1913 edition. The editors wrote, "Dr. Massey deserved great credit for having established single handedly, such a creditable little institution, which is deserving of the liberal patronage of the people of his community" (p. 278).

The ten-bed QHS was next door to Dr. Massey's home on West Windsor Street in Monroe. The 1913 *Annual report of the Board of Public Charities of North Carolina* stated that QHS was a private hospital owned by Dr. Massey, further noting that 100 patients had been admitted for medical and surgical treatment. Patients paid $1 to $1.50 a day for medical and nursing care, room, and board. Ninety-eight of the patients had improved or were cured and two died. Twenty-six were charity patients, unable to afford even the dollar a day costs of hospitalization. Three nurses were employed by the hospital (North Carolina Board, 1913). The hospital continued to grow. In 1915, Dr. Massey traveled to New York City to purchase electrical massage and x-ray equipment for QHS (North Carolina Board, 1915). Two hundred patients were treated in 1916, so Dr. Massey added four beds in 1917 for a total of 14 beds. The 1917 *Annual report of the Board of Public Charities of North Carolina* noted that an outpatient department had been organized and that "crippled and deformed children" were now being treated at QHS (North Carolina Board, 1917).

The 1930 census of Monroe lists Lillian Robertson as a nurse working at the QHS. Other nurses who worked at the facility include T. Beatrice Spellman and Carrie Marshall. The hospital continued to thrive, and another addition was completed in 1930. Unfortunately, in 1931, for reasons that have not been recorded, probably involving the national financial collapse known as the Great Depression, Dr. Massey gave the deeds to both his home and hospital to the City of Monroe in lieu of payment for paving assessments. By 1932, the town of Monroe allowed Dr. Massey to pay rent for his hospital as long as he was the one who operated it. When the hospital was put up for bid at a tax auction in 1939, Dr. Massey, the sole bidder, bought back QHS for $3,000 ("Dr. John Sherman Massey," 2016).

In 1942, during World War II, the U.S. Army opened Camp Sutton, a training camp and later Prisoner of War facility in Monroe. By this time, Dr. Massey was in his mid–70s and had developed kidney disease. He was no longer able to practice medicine, so he rented out rooms in the hospital to families of soldiers stationed at Camp Sutton. Dr. Massey died of kidney disease on May 12, 1946. A woman then bought the QHS building and ran it as the Dennis Motel for over ten years before it was abandoned. The building was so badly burned during a renovation in 1985 that it became unsalvageable and was demolished in 1988 ("John S. Massey," 2012).

Greensboro, Guilford County

The earliest known inhabitants of Guildford County were the Saura and Keyauwee people (Arnett, 1975). By the mid–1700s they had been replaced by white German, Quaker, and Scots-Irish settlers and enslaved Africans. Guildford County had fewer enslaved people—3,625 out of 29,056 people or 13 percent of the total population in 1860—than surrounding counties because Quaker teachings renounced slavery (Ptak, 2010). In fact, many of the area's Quakers were leaders in the Underground Railroad, helping enslaved people escape to free states (Coffin, 1968). Greensboro, the county seat of Guilford County, was home to a Confederate hospital and a Freedmen's Bureau hospital in the 1860s. The first modern hospital, St. Leo's, owned and operated by the Catholic Sisters of Charity, opened in 1905. There were 132 beds for white people and six for African Americans—three for men and three for women ("Sisters of Charity," 1931). In 1917, Dr. Wesley Long opened a large private hospital as a white-only institution (Long, 1972). When Moses Cone Hospital opened in 1953, administrators refused to hire any African American health professionals and "excludes all but a select few Negro patients, who are admitted on special conditions not applied to whites" (Sobeloff, 1963).

In the first decade of the 20th century most of the 15,000 African American residents of Guilford County who needed hospital services traveled by wagon over unpaved roads for 50 miles to Lincoln Hospital in Durham or 100 miles to Good Samaritan in Charlotte for surgery and hospital births. At the beginning of the 20th century, there were only a handful of Guilford County African American physicians to perform operations or assist with births in private homes (Phillips, 1993). Responding to this dire situation, in 1914, Dr. John Walter Vincent Cordice opened the first of three increasingly sophisticated hospitals for African Americans in Guildford County (Arnett, 1955).

Cordice Sanitarium

Dr. Cordice was born in the Caribbean country of St. Vincent to James Alex and Norz Anne Cordice on November 21, 1881. He moved to the United States to study medicine at Howard University/Freedmen's Hospital in Washington, D.C., graduating first in his class in 1913. Dr. Threlkield, the Dean of Howard Medical School, urged Dr. Cordice to move to Greensboro, North Carolina, the county seat of Guildford County, a medically underserved area with a large African American population ("Cordice, Dr. John," 2012). Following his mentor's advice, in 1914, Dr. Cordice opened the Cordice Sanitarium in an eight-bedroom house at 121 West McCullough Street in Greensboro. Soon after the institution opened, an article in the *Greensboro Daily News* reported:

> Passing up West McCullough Street from South Elm yesterday one's attention was attracted by automobiles belonging to certain families of the city standing in front of the Negro hospital. It was found that at this hospital many of the best and trusted servants are treated. They prefer to go out there because of the quietness, neatness and cleanliness of this hospital, where the patients are treated well and there is no caste prejudice. It was found that certain prominent families have sent their servants here for operations and treatment and paid for it because of the long and faithful service of the servant in the home. Out of 76 abdominal operations, not one percent has died ["Hospital for colored," 1915, p. 19].

A year later, on December 7, 1916, another article in the same newspapers, titled "The Colored Hospital" was published in the same newspaper:

> The hospital has been in operation here for about three years and the Negro doctors have successfully performed some very delicate abdominal operations, and this hospital has been of great service in curing, for sick servant girls who worked for white families and had no homes to go to while sick. Many of these cases have been charitable—in many such cases, however, the poor girls have not had the necessary night clothes while sick or clean clothes to get away from the hospital in when cured. For such emergencies, the hospital authorities have authorized the statement that if any warm-hearted people wish to give gowns, pajamas or anything else, they will gladly be accepted ["The Colored Hospital," 1916, p. 12].

Little more is known about this facility, but the need for a larger, more modern hospital soon became apparent (Phillips, 1996).

In May 1915, the Medical and Pharmaceutical Association of Guilford County, an African American professional organization, appointed a subcommittee of five physicians—Drs. Cordice, Sebastian, Stewart, McNair and Gerran—to work towards the establishment of a hospital for African Americans in Greensboro ("Decide to establish," 1915). In an appeal to the community that was published soon after the meeting, the committee discussed five reasons local people should support an African American hospital. They stressed that the number of available African American beds was insufficient to meet the need; the local hospital did not permit African American physicians to practice in the hospital, so patients were treated by unfamiliar white doctors instead of the physician of their choice; a recently enacted law prohibited white nurses from caring for African American patients so patients would be treated by less qualified white employees; racial pride would be enhanced by African Americans erecting and supporting their own hospital; and a modern hospital would greatly enhance the overall health of the African American population in the county ("Conducting campaign," 1915, p. 9).

Trinity Hospital

In 1918, Dr. Cordice joined forces with Dr. Charles Constantine Stewart and Dr. Simon Powell Sebastian to open the Trinity Hospital for Negroes in an 11-bedroom home on East Market Street in Greensboro (Philips, 1996). Dr. Stewart was born in Jamaica and was in Dr. Cordice's class at Howard Medical School. Dr. Sebastian was born in Antigua, another Caribbean Island, and initially came to Greensboro to teach at the Agricultural and Mechanical College (now North Carolina

Agricultural and Technical State University) in 1902. After a few years he decided to become a physician and graduated from Leonard Medical School in Raleigh in 1912 (Beckford, 2011). In addition to establishing Trinity Hospital, these three physicians, all from Caribbean islands, founded the Gate City Drug Company to provide medicine for their patients. Trinity Hospital was said to always be full, but was also describe as an "overcrowded and sub-standard" medical facility (Arnett, 1955; Greensboro Historical Museum, 1916, p. 1). An early mention of Trinity hospital was in the September 24, 1919, *Greensboro Daily News*. The newspaper noted, "Dr. J.W. Long and Dr. Parron Jarboe [well-regarded local white physicians] commended the work being done by the Negro hospital on East Market Street and thought it would be well to gender financial assistance to the institution..." ("Reports of committees," 1919, p. 9). A 1920 article in the local newspaper titled "Local Negro hospital needs financial aid" reported:

> The Colored Ministered Union ... calls the attention of the public to Trinity Hospital, an institution for the treatment of colored patients at 801 East Market Street, organized by the negro physicians of the city in 1919, and recommends it to the "generous public for aid." In placing this institution and its needs before the public, the Negro ministers of the city urge in particular that the Negro citizens rally to the institution and give it financial assistance, saying that by doing so they would be giving a tonic to their own racial self-respect ["Local Negro hospital," 1920, p. 8].

The daily fees at the hospital ranged from one dollar and fifty cents to two dollars a day. One hundred and twenty-five dollars had been donated to the hospital in its first eight months of operation. Costs not covered by paying patients and donations were borne by the physicians who managed the hospital. Ninety patients were treated the first year and "the mortality rate was almost nothing" ("Local Negro hospital," 1920, p. 8). Nurses employed at Trinity Hospital included Katie Corbett, head nurse, Susan Johnson, Nellie R. Calloway, Inez Donnell, Sallie Fitzgerald, and Mary L. Taylor (Greensboro Telephone Directories, 1920, 1921). Dr. Cordice moved to Aurora, North Carolina in 1918, accepting a position as a surgeon in the U.S. Public Health Service. After Dr. Cordice's departure, Drs. Sebastian and Stewart continued to operate Trinity Hospital. However, the 11-room, renovated house was inadequate to serve as a modern hospital in the 1920s (Arnett, 1955).

L. Richardson Hospital

In early January 1923, "a circular letter was sent out by a group of interested men to the colored people of Greensboro, calling them together ... [to get] a better understanding as to the needs of a hospital for the treatment of Negro patients" (Sebastian, 1930, p. 142). On January 20, 1923, a group of over 60 African American and White civic leaders held the charter meeting of the Greensboro Negro Hospital Association. The group launched a publicity and fundraising drive to erect a new, well-equipped hospital. Dr. Sebastian wrote an article about the founding of the new hospital. In his article he noted, "We began to call on our white friends, who have been friendly, disposed from the very beginning to aid us" (Sebastian, 1930, p. 142). Mrs. Mary Lynn Richardson, the widow of Lunsford Richardson, the founder of the Vicks Chemical Company, best known for creating Vicks VapoRub, quickly donated $50,000 to the hospital, which was later named L. Richardson Hospital in his honor. Mr. Richardson had a deep interest of the welfare of Greensboro's African American community and paid the salary of an African American public health nurse for Greensboro for several years in the 1910s (Greensboro Historical Museum, 2016; North Carolina Board, 1917). The Matheson-Wills-Benbow real estate company donated a four-and-a-half-acre site on East Washington Street for the hospital, and Mrs. Bertha Sternberger, widow of local textile industrialist and philanthropist Emmanuel Sternberger, donated $10,000 to equip an operating room and x-ray rooms in her late husband's honor (Elkins, 1969).

Construction began on the three-story, buff colored, fireproof, brick building in October 1926, and the first patient was admitted on May 18, 1927. The hospital was dedicated on May 27, 1927. The ceremony included a baby show, a track meet and a May Pole dance ("Baby show, track meet," 1927). Both the American Medical Association and the American College of Surgeons accredited the new hospital. There were 60 beds and four bassinets. Dr. Sebastian was the Chief of Staff, and physicians of both races admitted patients to the hospital and used the surgical and obstetrical facilities. Mrs. J. Reid was the first Director of Nursing and oversaw a nursing staff of five graduate nurses. She quickly started a three-year nursing school, which was accredited by the North Carolina Board of Nurse Examiners. Twenty young women enrolled in the first class in 1927. Reflecting the demanding curriculum and standards of the nursing school, only five of the initial 20 students graduated in 1930. One was Lillie Forte Berber, who worked at the Guildford County Health Department for 38 years, from her graduation in 1930 until her death in 1968 (Sebastian, 1930).

In 1930, Dr. Sebastian wrote about the hospitals early finances. When L. Richardson opened it was "without one penny for operating expenses and an indebtedness of $22,500 (incurred by virtue of the fact that many who pledged failed to make same good), but by careful buying, curtailing expenses and economical running of the hospital, this indebtedness has been reduced from $22,500 to $8,750" (Sebastian, 1930, p. 144). Financial help came in many forms during the Great Depression. The Duke Endowment paid $1.00 a day for each indigent patient's care. A Ladies Auxiliary was formed in 1929 to raise money and volunteer in the hospital for a myriad of duties. Mrs. J.E. Dellinger was its President. She reported, "This auxiliary is working in every department of the hospital and the results are splendid" (Sebastian, 1930, p. 144). The organization was formed "to perform acts of kindness to patients and nurses by visiting, giving flowers and reading

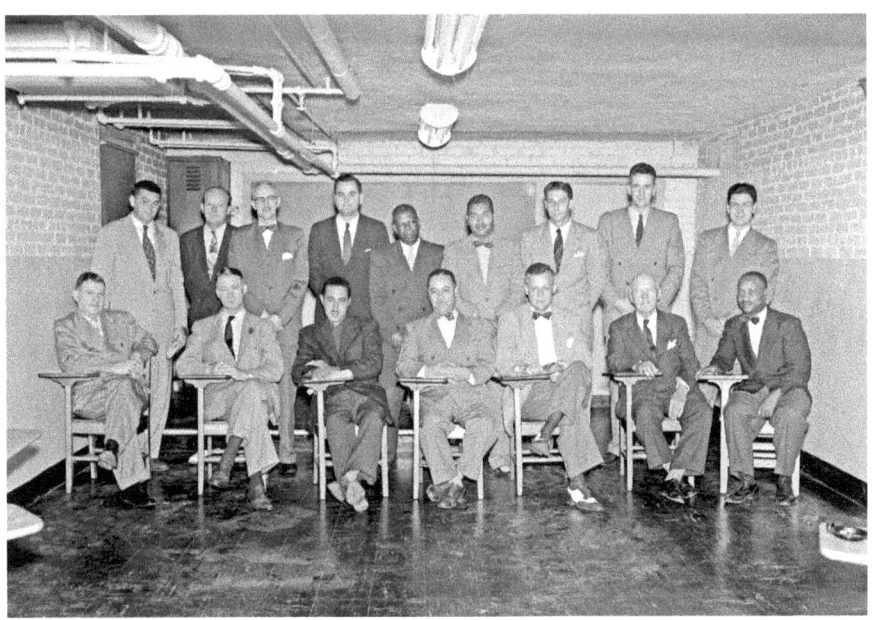

Doctors at L. Richardson Memorial Hospital, April 29, 1953 (copyright Carol W. Martin/Greensboro Historical Museum Collection).

materials, and to supply the needs the Board of Directors could not supply" (Elkin, 1969, p. 208).

The patient census grew each year and the facility expanded to meet the growing demand. In 1933, 832 patients were treated; of those, 363 were unable to financially contribute to their care, 289 paid a portion of their bills, and 180 were full-pay patients (L. Richardson, 1935). That number grew to 1,244 with 81 births in 1939 and a decade later, in 1948, over 3,000 patients were admitted. The growing number of patients seeking care necessitated expansions of the facility ("Negro hospital grows," 1940; Elkins, 1969). A $65,000 expansion in 1945–46 brought the total number of beds from 60 to 96. The obstetrical department added 12 beds and 17 bassinets ("Negroes to Have modern," 1945). Ten years later, in 1955, 5,325 patients spent 33,838 cumulative days in the hospital for a 92 percent occupancy rate. Dr. George Simkins remembered the hospital this way: "There would be beds in the hallways. You'd have to walk down a narrow path through the hallways without running into the beds, because it was so crowded" (Oral history, 1997). There were 627 major operations, 889 minor operations, 881 deliveries and 22,971 X-rays taken that year. Using monies from a Ford Foundation grant, the hospital fund balance and the federal Hill-Burton Act, in 1957 the hospital expanded to 110 beds and added new recovery and emergency rooms (Elkins, 1969).

In a 1963 legal case, titled *Simkins v. Moses H. Cone Memorial Hospital*, the U.S. 4th Circuit Court of Appeals ruled in a decision which was upheld by the U.S. Supreme Court, that Moses Cone and Wesley Long hospitals could no longer exclude African American patients or refuse to hire African American physicians and other health care professionals. The plaintiffs filed the suit on February 12, 1962, Abraham Lincoln's birthday, and the final decision was issued in November 1963. Despite this litigation, government and hospital leaders raised over $2,000,000 and erected a new L. Richardson Hospital, which admitted its first patients on June 13, 1966. The old building was converted to a nursing home (Reynolds, 1997). The new building continued to operate as city-owned, integrated, acute care hospital until 1985 when a group of seven private physicians bought the hospital and assumed its $3.1 million debt (McCauley, 1990). In Guilford County, at least token integration in local hospitals occurred as the result of the *Simkins* case months before the Civil Rights Act (CRA) of 1964 passed and years before Medicaid and Medicare made compliance with the CRA necessary to receive federal funds.

Oxford, Granville County

According to the Granville County Museum website:

> The land known today as Granville County was once the home of many Indian tribes, dominated mainly by the Tuscarora. After the Tuscarora War of 1711, settlers mostly from Virginia began to populate this area, attracted by the abundant game, well-watered woods, and rich land. By 1746, the area had a population sufficiently large enough to merit becoming an independent county, separating itself from Edgecombe County's western frontier [Thornton, 2007, p. 1].

In the years before the Civil War, Granville County, located in the northern central portion of the state, was a rich agricultural area, with over 11,000 enslaved people who produced high yields of tobacco and other cash crops, making local plantation owners very wealthy. By 1860, there were 1,121 free African Americans in the county (Hamrick, 2010). Oxford, the county seat, was both the cultural and governmental hub of the region, known for its several academies and colleges. Granville was one of the few counties in North Carolina to have a majority African American population in 1900. Of the 23,000 residents, 51 percent were African American and 49 percent were white ("Granville County History," 2016). Oxford became the home of the white Masonic Orphanage in 1838 and the tax-supported Colored Orphan Asylum of North Carolina in 1887. It was largely due to the needs of the African American orphans and the efforts of the staff at the orphanage that Oxford was home to two African American hospitals (Carlson & Brown, 1988).

On April 4, 1919, an interesting lot of items appeared in the Oxford newspaper, *The Public Ledger*. In a letter to the editor titled "A colored woman's plea for a hospital," Martha B. Spencer, an African American Registered Nurse and graduate of Lincoln Hospital School of Nursing in New York City, wrote, in part, "I have decided to establish a hospital in Oxford.... There was so much suffering among the people and the ravages of the Spanish influenza convinced me of the wisdom of such a step" (p. 1).

Another article published in the same edition reported on the progress of this endeavor:

> The colored people of Oxford have purchased the necessary land in "Cam Town" on which to erect a modern hospital. There are at present one or two wooden buildings on the lot, which are being fitted up and furnished for temporary use. Mrs. Spencer, a colored woman favorably known here, is in charge of the hospital. She has had considerable experience as a nurse and is said to be well qualified for the work.... It is understood that all of the colored people of means in the community are behind the hospital organization ["Funds available," 1919, p. 1].

A third related item, an announcement, in the same issue of the newspaper, publicized a public meeting regarding the hospital to be held April 6, 1919, at the First Baptist Church.

Apparently the hospital opened with a lot of community support. On the 4th of July 1919, several African American choirs competed in a competition at the courthouse to raise money for the hospital (Colored Folks, 1919). A month later, one hundred dollars were raised at another "entertainment" to benefit the hospital ("A nice donation," 1919). Sadly, a year after the hospital opened, a notice appeared in the April 9, 1920, *Oxford Public Ledger* announcing the sale of the hospital at a public auction. Nurse Martha Spencer defaulted on the mortgage she obtained the buy the hospital property. At the time of the sale, the property consisted of a hospital building and three tenant houses situated on five acres of land ("Sale of real estate," 1920). While very short-lived, the 1919–1920 hospital provided the groundwork for the successful establishment of the Susie Cheatham Hospital eight years later.

Susie Cheatham Memorial Hospital (SCMH)

Henry Cheatham, born into slavery on December 27, 1857, near Henderson, North Carolina, was a farmer, educator, politician, and hospital founder. He was elected as a Republican member of the United States House of Representatives and served from 1889 to 1893, one of only five African Americans elected to Congress from the South during the Jim Crow era. In the years around the turn of the 20th century, the North Carolina legislature enacted poll taxes (a tax on voting), literacy tests, and other means of disenfranchising African American voters. Cheatham lost his seat in Congress but was soon appointed Superintendent of the state-funded Colored Orphan Asylum in Oxford in 1907, a position he held for 28 years until his death in 1935 (Christopher, 1971).

Cheatham and his wife Laura had three children. Their daughter, Susie Clayton Cheatham, became a teacher at the orphanage and died of tuberculosis at age 23 in 1926. At that time, there were no sanitarium or hospital beds for African Americans in Granville County. Mr. Cheatham determined a hospital was needed to treat the health needs of the children and staff at the orphanage, as well as to serve the people in the surrounding communities. He spearheaded a drive to establish the Susie Cheatham Memorial Hospital. Mr. G.C. Shaw served as President of the Board of Directors and was joined by Mr. F.H.U. Edwards, Vice President, and Dr. Ellis E. Toney, secretary treasurer. Several local African American physicians pooled their money and, along with community donations, raised enough money to purchase the former home of John Young on Sycamore Street in Oxford and convert it into a 15-bed hospital with a well-equipped operating room ("Opening of Shaw," 1953). Equipment and supplies were donated or purchased, and the physicians alternated paying the mortgage on the building. A later description stated that the hospital "contained 25 beds and an assortment of furniture borrowed from citizens of the county" ("Erect race hospital," 1927, p. 1).

Ms. Augusta I. Grandy, RN, a 1926 graduate of St. Agnes Hospital School of Nursing in Raleigh, was hired as the Superintendent of Nursing. Other early nurses included St. Agnes graduates Betty Broadhurst (who later served as Superintendent), Rebecca Hennie, Annie L. Smith, and Practical Nurse Irene Bobbitt. Physicians using the hospitals were Dr. W.N. Thomas, Dr. G. Sam Watkins, Dr. R.L. Noblin, Dr. W.L. Taylor, Dr. S.M. Carrington, and Dr. E.E. Toney. The new hospital opened on May 4, 1927 (Barbee, 1927). Mr. Coley Barbee, in a letter to the editor in the September 20, 1927, edition of the *Public Ledger* reported that 162 patients were treated during the hospital's first few months of operation and of those, 159 were cured. Eighty-four successful operations had been performed in the first four and a half months of the hospital's existence. In 1929, 188 patients were admitted for a total of 2,635 days. The need for the hospital and its local acceptance were illustrated by the growth of both the number of patients and total bed days. By 1949, SCMH served 1,166 patients for a total of 4,793 days of care. Monthly operating costs in 1927 were $300 a month ("Need of Colored," 1950). Few if any patients had insurance at that time, and neither the state nor federal government had enacted programs to pay for hospitalization. Most of the patients were unable to cover their fees. Barbee (1927), in his letter wrote, "It has become necessary for the doctors to put in their own means that it [SCMH] may remain open. They have even, at times, out of their own resources, furnished the salary of the superintendent and her assistants" (n.p.). The county did pay for a few charity cases each year, and by 1932, the hospital was receiving annual donations from the Duke Endowment, the philanthropic arm of the Duke Energy Company. In 1932, the Duke Endowment gave the hospital $1 a day for charity care for a total of $1,542.

In 1938, the new white-only Granville Hospital was built with public funds. African American citizens were assured that adequate, tax-supported hospital facilities would be provided for them as well, as the new Granville Hospital had no designated "Negro beds" (McGhee, 2014). A old school property was designated as the site for a new African American hospital in Oxford ("School property." 1938). It would be another 14 years until a new hospital building was erected.

After World War II, improvements in surgical techniques, the development of new medications, and the advances in laboratory testing and body imaging made the SCMH obsolete. An article in the *Public Ledger* described the SCMH building as "a frame building, which has become overcrowded. Lacking a central heating plant, it is poorly designed and wholly inadequate for use as a modern hospital" ("Building fund," 1945, n.p.). There was no delivery suite or pediatric unit. The facility was also a fire hazard, and only a reprieve granted by the state fire marshal allowed the building to remain in use. No repairs, additions, or changes that might prolong the use of the hospital were permitted by state agencies ("Need of Colored hospital," 1950). Adding to the hospital's difficulties was the discontinuation, in 1949, of a $1-a-day payment for charity care provided by state funds due to the hospital being owned by a self-perpetuating Board of Trustees rather than by a public entity ("Susie Cheatham," 1949).

A committee of local African American citizens, led by Dr. Toney, launched a drive to raise $75,000 for a new hospital ("Building fund,"1945, n.p.). Seven local physicians each donated $500 to the fundraising campaign ("Doctors give," 1945). By 1950, enough money had been raised to purchase nine acres of land for the new hospital's site. The SCMH Board of Trustees offered the land to the county to build an African American hospital. A successful bond referendum passed on September 16, 1950, funding a new 30-bed, one-story brick hospital for African Americans along with a new 24-bed addition to the Granville Hospital for whites. The new African American hospital was named Shaw Memorial Hospital, honoring Dr. G.C. Shaw, the late educator and SCMH Board member (McGhee, 2014).

Shaw Memorial Hospital (SMH)

The new $400,000, county-owned Shaw Memorial Hospital opened on January 31, 1953. It was described as an "ultra-modern hospital, fitted with the latest medical and surgical equipment for the best possible treatment and for the maximum comfort of the patients" ("Shaw Hospital," 1952, n.p.). In addition to 30 beds, there were two operating rooms, one designated as an emergency operating room, an X-ray department, a laboratory, and a kitchen that could serve 150 people daily. African American and white physicians on staff at the new hospital included Drs. W.L. Taylor, W.N. Thomas, E.E. Toney, R.L. Noblin, S.M. Carrington, R.W. Taylor, Ballard Norwood, J.C. Elliott, J.S. Bradsher, Sam Daniel, E.L. Clay, and Joseph Colson. Registered Nurses who worked at SMH included Miss Ora Lee Person, Superintendent, Mrs. Elizabeth Davis Sheppard, Miss Betty S. Broadhurst, and Mrs. Annie L. Winston. Practical Nurses included Mrs. Estelle Virginia Heard, Miss Lucinda Baskerville, and Mrs. Irene Bobbitt ("Shaw Hospital," 1953).

Granville was one of the last counties to desegregate its hospitals. Shaw Memorial Hospital served the county's and surrounding African American communities for 14 years. In 1967, four years after the *Simkins v. Moses H. Cone* court decision, three years after the 1964 Civil Rights Act and only under threat of losing Medicare payments from the federal government, did Granville Hospital open its doors to all of the citizens of Granville County.

Smithfield, Johnston County

Furlonge Hospital, 1929–1951

After the Tuscarora people were displaced by war and disease in the early 1700s, many white settlers and enslaved people moved from Virginia and Maryland into the area now known as Johnston County. The county was created in 1746 and, during the time covered in this book, was rural, encompassing several small towns including Smithfield, Selma, and Benson. In 1860, the county population was composed of 10,656 whites, 4,916 enslaved people, and 195 free African Americans. Almost all of the eligible white men residing in Johnston County served in the Confederate army, about 1,500 total. Until the mid–1900s, most county residents worked in the production and/or sale of its two main agricultural products: cotton and tobacco (Lassiter, Lassiter, & Lassiter, 2004). African Americans comprised between 21 percent and 25 percent of the county's population in the decades around the turn of 20th century ("Johnston County History," 2016).

The early hospitals in Johnston County were white-only institutions. Dr. Charles Furlonge opened his clinic in 1929, providing the first in-patient, overnight care for African Americans in the region (K.T. Johnson, personal communication, March 29, 2016). Before that time, the closest African American hospital was St. Agnes Hospital in Raleigh, a 30–50-mile trip over unpaved roads. When Dr. Furlonge decided to open his practice in Johnston County, medical care for the county's 12,000 African Americans was badly needed (Fisher & Buckley, 2016).

Charles William Furlonge was born to Octavious and Ann Maria Furlonge on the Caribbean Island of Montserrat on February 14, 1887. He decided as a young man to become a physician and serve the poor. He entered Shaw University in Raleigh in 1909, where he completed two years of college courses and four years of medical training at Leonard Medical School. Furlonge graduated with his MD degree in 1914. After graduation he became the first physician to enter the internship program at St. Agnes Hospital in Raleigh (Hulth, 1963). In 1916, Dr. Furlonge was on his way to Dunn, North Carolina, to open an office, but a winter storm caused him to stop in Johnston County and he decided to stay. He opened his first office in 1915 in Selma where he "almost starved to death for 12 months" (Hulth, 1963, p. 1). Soon he settled in Smithfield where he would practice medicine for the next 53 years (Heritage of Johnston, 1985).

Dr. Furlonge stayed up to date in medical and surgical practices by participating in annual continuing education programs. For seventeen summers he attended two-week clinics at the Medical College at Richmond, Virginia. He took special courses in pediatrics at the Saluda Clinic near Hendersonville for seven summers. Additionally, Dr. Furlonge spent three weeks for six summers in courses offered by the Bowman Gray School of Medicine in Winston-Salem (Hulth, 1963).

The Heritage of Johnston County recounts Furlonge's struggling early years of medical practice: "With no means of transportation, he went by foot or train, and sometimes neighbors would loan him a horse and buggy.... Dr. Furlonge accepted vegetables, meat, eggs or whatever farmers had in lieu of money" (Heritage of Johnston, 1985, p. 221). One writer described Dr. Furlonge's dedication to the people of Johnston County as

> a man on call 24 hours a day, seven days a week, traveling to the side of the sick and dying through the frigid blasts of winter and the stifling heat of summer, in the blast of noon sun and darkness of post-midnight hours [Cannon, 1983, p. B-1].

In 1929, Dr. Furlonge opened the first African American hospital in Johnston County. He built his first examination table by hand because he did not have enough money to purchase a new one and pay its freight costs. Children from each of the 22 local African American schools donated money for the hospital. New Bethel School students raised a total of 64 cents, while students at Wilson's Mills School donated nine dollars ("Negroes report," 1926). An article in the January 15, 1929, edition of the *Smithfield Herald* describes the hospital as "An institution that is destined to be a beacon light among the Negroes of Johnson County pointing the way to better health and sanitation" ("Negro hospital opens its doors," 1929, p. 1). The brick and concrete building on Massey Street, erected at a cost of approximately $6,000, housed a "well-lighted, modernly equipped operating room with a small room for a sterilizer," a maternity ward, a doctor's office, kitchen, dining room, a 10-bed ward, five private patient rooms, and a bath on the first floor ("Negro hospital opens its doors," 1929, p. 1). The second floor had three rooms for the nursing staff. Mrs. Mary A. Moore, RN, graduate of Harlem Hospital in New York City, was the head nurse and was assisted by two or three nursing students. Mrs. Flora Smith, of Smithfield, was a nurse at the hospital for over 25 years. Local leaders and churches supported the hospital. Among the many donations were six pillows from the African American Smithfield Presbyterian Church. The African American Presbyterian church in nearby Benson gave sheets, pillow cases, and blankets. An association of Smithfield African American women donated a heatrola to heat the operating room and another unnamed source supplied an icebox ("Negro hospital opens its doors," 1929).

Dr. Furlonge's Hospital served the community for 22 years until Johnston Memorial Hospital (JMH) opened in 1951. In the beginning, JMH was strictly segregated with white and Negro wards. However, in an arrangement unusual for the times, Dr. Furlonge was allowed hospital and operating room privileges at the new hospital (Cannon, 1983). Johnston Memorial Hospital fully integrated in the 1960s. As racial attitudes changed in the late 1960s and 1970s, Dr. Furlonge received many honors and awards before his death in 1972. In 1970, he was chosen as the "Distinguished Citizen" of the area by the local Chamber of Commerce. Other awards included being honored as a "dedicated humanitarian" by Smithfield's First Missionary Baptist Church and "Parent of the Year" by the Johnston Central School for his free physicals and support of various sports teams. In addition, a road in Smithfield was named Furlonge Drive in his honor ("Ministered to the community," 1970, p. 6). In addition to his busy medical practice, Dr. Furlonge was active in many civic affairs. He served on the Board of Trustees of both the Johnston Memorial Hospital and Fayetteville State University, was a member of the Smithfield School Board Advisory Committee, the Smithfield Housing Authority, and the Johnston County Committee for Mental Health. Dr. Furlonge was also involved in many professional organizations, including the American Medical Association (white) and the National Medical Association (African American), the NC Medical Society (white) and the Old North State Medical Society (African American), and the Johnston County Medical Association ("Dr. C.W. Furlonge," 1972).

Dr. Furlonge's exemplary work and commitment is representative of the 13 physicians who filled a deep void by opening health care facilities in unserved areas of North Carolina. Despite personal financial risks, long hours as solo practitioners meeting the overwhelming needs of thousands of vulnerable patients, and overt racism practiced by their fellow white physicians, Dr. Furlonge and his colleagues overcame the challenges. They could have practiced in northern or western states where there were no Jim Crow segregation laws; they could have practiced in cities where they could share the responsibilities of providing healthcare with other African American physicians. Instead, a small number of physicians, including Dr. Furlonge, took it upon themselves to build hospitals, clinics, and sanatoria in rural areas, providing care to perhaps the most neglected citizens of North Carolina.

Gastonia, Gaston County

Until the mid–1700s, the area now known as Gaston County was inhabited by Catawba and Cherokee people. They were driven out by Scots-Irish, Pennsylvania Dutch, and English settlers. By 1860, Gaston County's population totaled 9,310 people of which 7,009 were white. African Americans made up about one quarter of the county's population; 2,199 were enslaved and 102 were free (Ptak, 2010). Soil conditions made corn, with its byproduct of whiskey, the main cash crop in Gaston County before the Civil War. Farming gave way to industrialization, particularly textile manufacturing, as the primary economic force in the area in the post-bellum era (Ragan, 2010). In 1908, the city of Gastonia, the county seat, opened City Hospital. It only admitted white patients and did not extend practice privileges to African American physicians. The closest African American hospital was Good Samaritan in Charlotte, a ten to 40-mile distance from towns in Gaston County.

Dr. Erwin's Hospital/ The Colored Hospital, 1920–1937

Dr. Herbert Jones Erwin, Jr., born in 1879 in Morganton, graduated from Leonard Medical School in Raleigh, North Carolina, in 1908. He moved to Gastonia and began his medical practice (Beckford, 2011). At that time, there were few African American physicians west of Charlotte, so he treated patients from a wide area in western North Carolina and northern South Carolina. He was described as "of a sunny and genial disposition. He carried with him at all times an atmosphere of friendliness and good cheer that was an unfailing boost to the spirits of anyone who happened to be ill" (Jeffers, 1946, p. 1). No local hospital would allow him practice privileges, so most of his work was performed in patient homes. Few patients could afford to pay for medical services, so Dr. Erwin accepted food and useful items in exchange for medical care (Gaston County Museum, n.d.).

Dr. Erwin and his wife, Daisy Blair Erwin, traveled through the region, making appearances at churches, fraternal organizations, and other large assemblies soliciting funds for an African American hospital in Gastonia. Others joined in their efforts, and Dr. Erwin became the

President of the Board of Trustees of the hospital movement. In addition to several concerts and church suppers, Dr. Erwin arranged a magic show and oyster roast to raise funds for the new hospital ("Colored hospital nearing," 1919). A newspaper story noted, "The colored citizens of Gaston County are now on their second rally in the interest of the Colored hospital and the thermometer of enthusiasm and determination is rising rapidly, reaching the 100th degree" ("Colored hospital movement," 1919). The Gaston County commissioners contributed $250 to the hospital fund ("Commissioners give," 1920). Hundreds of local African American citizens donated $500 in fifty-cent, $1, and $2 increments ("Colored hospital is soon," 1919). A story in the November 29, 1919, *Gastonia Gazette* reported that $4,000 of the needed $6,000 had been raised and that a two-story, brick building with central heating was being erected. The cornerstone was laid with a ceremony that included music and barbeque ("Colored hospital," 1919).

Dr. Erwin announced the opening of the hospital in an item in the *Gastonia Gazette* on April 30, 1920. He invited all citizens of Gaston County to an open house and asked for donations of "soaps, washing powders, gowns, towels, sheets, pillows, blankets, spreads, cooking and eating utensils" ("Public opening," 1920, p. 1). Dr. Erwin—along with two African American physicians, Dr. W. Perry Carter and Dr. Thomas H. Williston—constituted the facility's medical staff. White physicians James M. Sloan and Charles Glenn used the hospital's operating room to perform surgery on their African American patients. In 1920, physicians from the North Carolina State Board of Health held a free clinic to screen for tuberculosis at Dr. Erwin's Hospital ("Anti-tuberculosis," 1920). The number of people seeking hospital services became greater than the space could easily accommodate. Overcrowded conditions in the hospital were remembered this way: "Years ago the 35 bed hospital was operating at capacity or overflowing" and as "35 beds stacked one on top of the other" (Jimison, 1962, p. A-9). Some of the early nurses were Cora Johnson, Head Nurse, Daisy McWrath, and Mattie Rabb ("The earliest," n.d.). Hundreds of patients were treated at Dr. Erwin's Hospital over almost two decades. In time, the furniture, linens, and equipment became outdated. During the Great Depression of the 1930s, donations to the hospital declined, as did the number of patients who were able to pay their full bills.

Gaston County Colored Hospital (GCCH), 1937–1966

Due to overcrowding at Dr. Erwin's hospital, as well as a need for more modern facilities, on November 16, 1937, the new Gaston County Colored Hospital (GCCH), a one-story, brick hospital opened across the street from Dr. Erwin's Hospital. The City of Gastonia donated six acres of land valued at $7,500, the Duke Endowment donated $12,500, and the Gaston County Commissioners donated $10,000. An additional $18,500 was raised from private donations (Gaston, 1946). The hospital was owned and operated by Gaston County, and all of the hospital's Board of Trustees, administrators, and nursing supervisors were white ("Gastonia Negro Hospital," 1954). Gaston County Colored Hospital had 19 beds composed of four four-bed wards and three private rooms. The new hospital boasted an operating room, an emergency room, an x-ray room, a kitchen, a waiting room, and two bedrooms for nurses (Williams, 1950).

In 1937, GCCH's first year of operation, 80 patients were treated. A report published in 1947 detailing the hospital's first ten years showed a total of 1,429 patients had been treated, for 29,995 bed days. Fees were $4 per day for a bed in a ward and $5 a day for a private room. The average census was 14 patients a day. In 1946, 685 patients were treated at the hospital. Expenses for the year were $1,439.55 and income was $1,389.63, leaving a deficit of $49.92. The state of North Carolina provided $1 a day for charity cases (Alexander, 1947).

A 1950 expansion, funded by a grant from the Ford Foundation, added 16 beds, a new operating room, a maternity ward, a nursery, new furniture, a kitchen, a waiting room, a storage area, and two rooms for nurses. Community members and organizations donated needed items to the hospital ("Hospital for Negroes," 1951). In 1954, the Women's Civic Club donated 36 place settings of china and silver to the hospital and the Ushers Union gave an oxygen tent ("Silver and China," 1954; "Ushers Union," 1954). Hazel Neely Boyd, Virginia Trollinger, and Eva Spring were the three Registered Nurses caring for patients. They were assisted by three practical nurses, including Marie McKinley and Eugenia Blair. The hospital averaged caring for 25 patients a day ("Hospital for Negroes," 1951).

By the mid–1950s, financial problems plagued GCCH. In 1957, rates were raised to $7 a day for a bed in a ward, $8 a day for a semi-private room, and $10 a day for a private room ("Rates raised," 1957). An article in *The Gastonia Gazette* informed its readers that the GCCH was facing "staggering losses" ("Negro institution losing money," 1959, p. 9). Fifty percent of its patients were certified charity patients. These cases accounted for 2,328 bed days. The hospital spent more than a dollar per day on charity patients than it received in subsidies, meaning it lost money on every charity patient. Gaston County subsidized each charity patient at a rate of $10 per day. In addition, the Duke Endowment contributed $1 per day and the Kate B. Reynolds Fund contributed another 85 cents a day for each charity patient. Another 28 percent of the hospital's patients were considered "total losses" because they could not contribute to their bills, nor were they certified as charity cases and thus were not entitled to the subsidies. After some of the food suppliers to the hospital refused to bring more meat because they were not getting paid, the Gaston County Commissioners had an emergency meeting and increased their subsidy to $14 a day ("County ups," 1959). This kept the hospital viable but not operating optimally.

Until 1962 when a $30,000 expansion allowed for the addition of a laboratory and an x-ray department, African American patients had to travel several miles to Gaston Memorial Hospital for these services (Jimison, 1962, p. A-9). White leaders of Gaston County did not anticipate racial segregation's rapid demise. Due to court cases and changing legislation that ordered all hospitals to racially integrate just a year after the 1962 expansion of GCCH, Gaston County officials integrated Gaston Memorial Hospital in 1963, converting GCCH to a nursing home in 1966 ("Community hospital," 1966).

Wilmington, New Hanover County

Community Hospital, 1920–1967

Very little is known about the earliest inhabitants of the southeastern coastal area of North Carolina, not even the tribal names, language or larger affiliations. The so-called Cape Fear Indians, named by settlers and scholars for the largest river in the area, were exterminated by the early 1700s due to war, disease and Native slavery (Hotz, 2007). At the eve of the Civil War, in 1860, New Hanover County had slightly more African American than white residents. Of the 21,715 people living in the county, 10,617 were white, 10,332 enslaved, and 766 were free African Americans (Ptak, 2010).

By the turn of the 20th century, Wilmington, the county seat of New Hanover County and a port city near the mouth of the Cape Fear River, was North Carolina's largest city. Its population of around 30,000 was approximately one-third African American and two-thirds white. This was a time of significant racial strife. After the election of 1898, in which the majority of city offices were won by African American and sympathetic white Republican men, about 2,000 white men murdered dozens of African Americans, burned the offices of the African American newspaper and expelled at least 20 specifically targeted individuals from Wilmington, putting them, at gunpoint, on northbound trains. Some 2,100 other residents, mostly African Americans, left the city in the following days and weeks in a mass exodus. The event is widely described as the only successful coup d'etat in American history (Cecelski & Tyson, 1998).

A 1920 editorial in the *Wilmington Star*, praising the efforts of African Americans to establish a hospital, harkened back to the 1898 massacre. It read in part, "as late as 1898, when he [the African American] was brought to his senses, when he was compelled to face the long task of finding himself, of becoming through industry, thrift and self-respect a dependable, competent, developing member of society ... the desire for a negro hospital is the symbol of an aspiration which ought to be fulfilled" ("The Negro Hospital," 1920).

Although Wilmington had been home to both the U.S. Army General Hospital for Colored Troops during the Civil War and a Freedman's Bureau hospital during Reconstruction, the earliest civilian hospitals, Lane Hospital, which operated from 1875 through 1900 and the tax-exempt James Walker Memorial Hospital (JWMH), which opened in 1902, were established as white-only institutions. No accommodations for African American patients, even those with life-threatening emergencies, were available in the county (Medical Society, 1977). African American physicians were forced to treat patients in their homes, often under adverse conditions. Dr. Frank Avant, a 1908 Leonard Medical School graduate, arrived in Wilmington in 1909. He described his early experiences practicing medicine in patient homes since no area hospitals allowed him to treat patients:

> Having no hospital connections, I was terribly shocked when I had to deliver babies in Brown's Alley, in Love's Alley, under the most unsanitary conditions,

and operating on a small kitchen table or sitting in a very low chair beside a low bed to operate [Medical Society, 1977, p. 48].

On June 21, 1905, James Walker Hospital opened its "Colored Annex" named the Sprunt Ward. Dr. Hubert Eaton described the facility in his autobiography.

> Walker Memorial maintained approximately 25 beds for Negro patients in a ward that had but two toilets and was in a building separated completely from the main hospital. To reach the operating room, delivery room, X-ray department, or any of the hospital's other special treatment facilities, the patients had to be wheeled or walked, unsheltered, about 30 yards, exposing them to all kinds of weather. Black physicians were barred from practicing in the Annex [Eaton, 1984, p. 53].

Mrs. Helen Lofton, an African American nurse who gave birth at JWMH twice in the late 1950s was interviewed in 2004 by Ms. LuAnn Mims. She recalled the Sprunt Ward this way:

> MIMS: How was it subdivided? It surely wasn't just an open ward, was it?
> LOFTON: Well, yes 'cause I can remember when you walked in the door, when you first went in, I think there was a birthing room over here on the right and then you walked back a little ways and I think on either side were maybe rooms with maybe 2, 3, no ... 4 patients in them. Then you would go further back and there was a ward, what they call a ward and they were like cubicles because you could either go left or right.
> I think the women were on this side and the men were on that side because I remember being back there in a cubicle in this ward. I remember they took me up front to deliver and then I went back there. So everything was in that one annex.
> MIMS: It's amazing that they were able to keep like wound infections away from the new moms.
> LOFTON: I know, isn't that scary now? That was scary.
> MIMS: Especially with new babies. Where were the new babies kept?
> LOFTON: Where was the nursery, I can't remember now, I think there was still a little area ... but we were all packed in that annex. Now that I have been in nursing and what not and I think about how all of us were just in there together like that, it sends me into a tailspin [Lofton, 2004, pp. 9–10].

Under these dire conditions, the seven physicians making up the Wilmington branch of the Old North State Medical Society—Drs. Austin, Avant, Bowens, Burnett, Chestnut, Kay and Parris—discussed founding their own hospital. Several disputes arose among the physicians, and several withdrew from the planning committee. However, other members of the community felt the urgent need for an African American hospital. Together, the Rev. W.H. Moore, the Rev. A.J. Wilson,

Julius A. Murray, David Bryant, Thomas Hooper, Dr. John Kay and Dr. Foster Burnette chartered and became the first Trustees of the Community Hospital (Avant, 1939). The trustees, with donations from both African American and White supporters, purchased the Niestlie Drug Store, a two-story, white, wood-frame building at 415 North 7th Street ("In training," 2004). After remodeling, it opened as Community Hospital in January 1921. The first floor housed the reception area, laboratories, doctor's offices, the X-ray room, bathrooms, nursing quarters, the dining room, the kitchen and a few patient rooms. Upstairs were the operating room, sterilizing room, private rooms, two wards and the bathrooms. An item in the local newspaper reported the hospital staff hoped to add an addition for a nursery, noting:

> When the hospital opened three weeks ago, new babies were placed in one of the rooms in the main part of the building, but when the number increased to twenty, the wee occupants made such as fuss that they disturbed the regular patients and had to be sent home ["Community hospital," 1921, p. 8].

The same article asked the public to donate screens for the windows to prevent mosquitoes from entering the building ("Community hospital," 1921). The building used steam heat and had electricity and running water. Dr. John Kay, Dr. Foster Burnette and registered nurses Mabel Coe, a graduate of St. Agnes Hospital in Raleigh, and Georgia C. King were the first full-time staff members. By 1921, four young women were in nurses training at the hospital, although the program had yet to be accredited (Avant, 1939). In 1922 the North Carolina Legislature appropriated $13,000 to support the hospital ("The Community Hospital," 1923).

An article in the September 18, 1922, *Wilmington Morning Star* reported on a visit made to Community Hospital by two white Chamber of Commerce officials. They stated that everything was clean and orderly, and that the nurses were "very polite, efficient and much interested in the cases" ("Chamber secretary," 1922, p. 8). During the week the Chamber officials visited, 20 patients were hospitalized and 17 major operations were performed. The Chamber visitors were surprised to find that patients could settle their accounts with "donations of foodstuffs such as chickens, eggs etc." ("Chamber secretary," 1922, p. 8).

In 1922, Miss Salome Taylor joined the staff as Superintendent of the Hospital and Director of the School of Nursing. Her contributions were invaluable to the hospital and to the lives of over 250 African

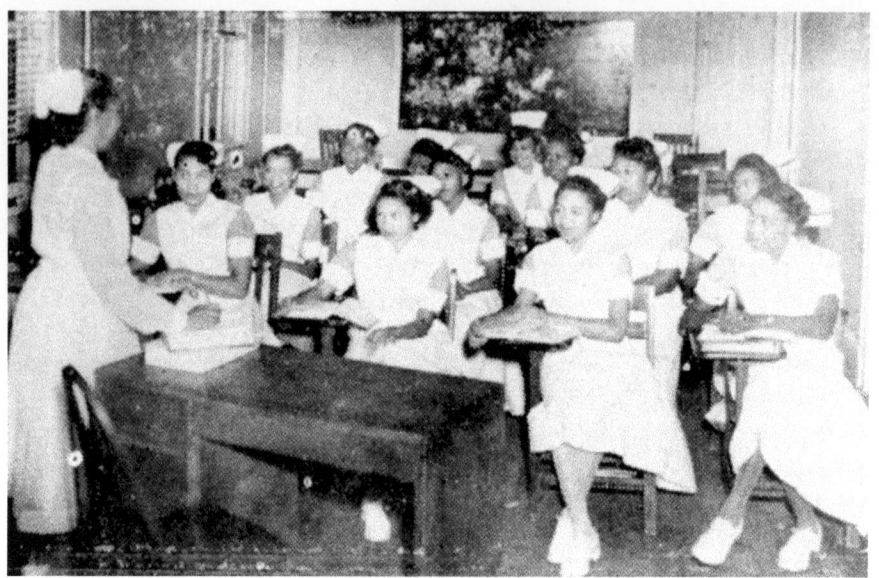

Nursing students in a classroom at Community Hospital, Wilmington, from *Bulletin of the Community Hospital School of Nursing*, 1960–61 (Dr. Hubert A. Easton, Sr., Manuscript Collection, William Madison Randall Library Special Collections, University of North Carolina–Wilmington, Wilmington, North Carolina).

American nurses she taught and supervised from 1922 to 1950 (Steelman, 2011). One of highest priorities for Taylor was upgrading the nursing training program to become an accredited school of nursing whose graduates could sit for the state Registered Nurse examinations. From 1920 to 1927, students in the nursing program learned through on-the-job training and occasional classes from the staff nurses and physicians. A news item detailing the 1924 nursing graduation exercises was published in *The Pittsburgh Courier.* The graduates received pins and "Dr. Farthing made some very touching remarks on the good work of the hospital and the good it has done for the community" ("Wilmington, N.C.," 1924). Upon graduation students earned the titles "graduate nurse" or "trained nurse" but because the program was not accredited, could not become Registered Nurses. Their career opportunities were largely limited to working as private duty nurses or in local hospitals.

The Community Hospital School of Nursing opened in 1927 and replaced the fragmented apprenticeship-type program that preceded it. Coursework was difficult and comprehensive including chemistry and pathology (Godwin, 2000). The first class of three nurses, Ruth Hines, Isler and Simmons, graduated in 1930. By the 1940s the school received an "A" rating from the North Carolina Board of Nurses, and the school was selected for participation in the U.S. Cadet Nursing Program by the U.S. Army. At least 17 Community Hospital nursing students were accepted into that program, committing themselves to serve the nursing needs of the armed forces during World War II (Ancestry.com, 2011). In 1963, Wilmington mayor O.O. Allsbrook proclaimed May 12 (Florence Nightingale's birthday and National Nurses Day) "Salome Taylor Day" to recognize her contributions to the people of the city ("Salome Taylor," 1963). The hospital initiated a residency program for African American physicians; the first doctor to participate was Dr. Daniel Roane in 1938 followed by Dr. Samuel Jones Grey the next year (Avant, 1939).

The Great Depression of the 1930s damaged the hospital's financial status, but the hospital remained open. Some financial relief came by the mid–1930s when the Duke Endowment began providing a dollar a day for each patient classified as needing indigent care (Eaton, 1965). Numerous fund-raisers from concerts to bake sales were held to support the hospital. Nursing Superintendent Taylor's salary was cut in half; she lived in the hospital and ate from the hospital kitchen during these years. Physicians were forced to take on many duties. They performed surgery, provided post-operative care for patients, ran the X-ray room and laboratories and taught in the nursing school. At times, even hospital trustees took turns firing the furnace and doing janitorial work. Despite these obstacles, in the twelve years between 1927 and 1939, Community hospital physicians admitted 6,237 patients for a total of 64,041 days of care, performed 1,129 major and 2,144 minor surgeries and attended 766 births (Avant, 1939).

By the late 1930s, the hospital needed a larger and more modern physical plant. Patients were sleeping on mattresses on the floor and on operating room tables when no surgeries were taking place. Dr. Foster Burnette, the driving force behind the hospital, sometimes feared that visitors had come to seize equipment or close the hospital because of the hospital's mounting debts. Local residents helped meet the need for better African American hospital facilities by passing a bond issue in 1939. Those funds, coupled with $110,000 from the federal Works Progress Administration program were enough to erect a new brick, three-story Community Hospital located on the corner of 11th and Church streets. Capacity doubled with beds for 40 patients. Due to the nature of funding for the new hospital, ownership was transferred from the private Board of Directors to the City of Wilmington and New Hanover County. The hospital earned accreditation from the American Hospital Association and the American College of Surgeons (Godwin, 2000).

During World War II, Wilmington was a major ship-building center for the U.S. Navy. The population of the town doubled; many of the new residents were African American. The federal government again provided money for a 56-bed addition to Community Hospital in 1943, bringing the total bed count to 96. Despite all of these improvements, Community Hospital still lacked the ability to provide many services, notably care for contagious disease and psychiatric illness (Godwin, 2000). No other major renovations occurred before Community Hospital closed in 1967 (Eaton, 1984).

Because of the ban on African American physicians treating their patients at the white, public James Walker Hospital, and because of the disparities in funding, staffing and equipment between Community Hospital and James Walker Hospital, in 1957, Dr. Hubert Eaton, physician, civil rights activist and gifted amateur tennis player, led several of his fellow local African American physicians in a lawsuit to racially integrate James Walker Memorial Hospital. They lost their case (Mangus, 2015). Six years later the *Simkins v. Moses H. Cone* case was decided, and within another year the Civil Rights Act of 1964 was enacted. Both Community and James Walker Hospital were aging and needed major maintenance and upgrading to meet ever-increasing standards from the American Hospital Association. Instead of putting money into renovating two aging hospitals, voters in New Hanover County passed a bond issue to erect one new state-of-the-art facility. The new New Hanover Memorial Hospital opened on June 14, 1967. Patients and staff from both the James Walker Memorial Hospital and Community Hospital moved into the new hospital without incident. For almost 50 years, Community Hospital provided care to thousands of poor, sick and vulnerable people. The founders and leaders of Community Hospital were honored by a plaque placed in the 1939 Community Hospital building. Its words apply to all of the employees and supporters of the hospital throughout its existence, "Because they loved their fellow man they gave liberally in service and substance that their dreams for the relief of suffering humanity might become a reality" (Eaton, 1965, p. 78).

Mount Olive, Wayne County

Rivera Clinic, 1920s–1965

Wayne County, a largely agricultural county is located in the coastal plains region of eastern North Carolina. The county includes many large farms that produced high yields of cotton and tobacco in the antebellum era as well as several small towns including Seven Springs, Mount Olive and Goldsboro. The earliest known inhabitants of Wayne County were the Saponi and Tuscarora people. Later, colonists from the British Isles and enslaved Africans settled the region and the indigenous people were decimated by war and disease. In 1860, the county's population consisted of 8,721 whites, 5,451 enslaved people and 734 free African Americans (Ptak, 2010). By 1900 the county's population was 31,056 with 17,887 white citizens and 13,169 African Americans. Although the county was home to North Carolina's large, tax-supported, segregated, psychiatric hospital for African Americans, only one small general clinic in the town of Mount Olive offered hospital care for local African American residents.

The county's first general hospital, Wayne County Memorial Hospital opened in 1896 in Goldsboro and admitted only white patients. Wayne County was also home to a little-known and poorly documented hospital for African Americans in the small farming community of Mount Olive. The Rivera Clinic was founded by Dr. Tomas Monte Rivera in 1916. Dr. Rivera was born on December 29, 1889, to Jose and Ramona Rivera in Arecibo, Puerto Rico. His Hispanic origins seemed to blur, even confuse, the binary color line in North Carolina where people were legally classified as either white or colored. Dr. Rivera attended high school in Puerto Rico, and after graduating from Tuskegee Institute in Alabama, attended Leonard Medical School in Raleigh in 1911–1912. He graduated from Meharry Medical School in Nashville, Tennessee, in 1915 ("Dr. Thomas Monte Rivera," 1953). He volunteered for service in World War I, but there is no record that he was called into action. Dr. Rivera completed residencies at both King County Hospital in Brooklyn, New York and St. Agnes Hospital in

Raleigh, North Carolina, before he moved to Mount Olive in 1916. There, he opened the wood frame, 10-bed, Rivera Clinic. At that time, the closest hospital that would admit African Americans was 40 miles away in Wilson, North Carolina. Dr. Rivera treated both African American and white patients in his office ("Dr. Rivera's Clinic," 1930). In days without paved roads, and at a time few white people and fewer African Americans owned automobiles, a 40-mile wagon trip over unpaved roads caused additional pain and suffering for those already needing medical care.

Dr. Rivera practiced medicine in Mount Olive for 48 years and was known throughout eastern North Carolina. Patients came from as far away as Wilmington on a regular basis. Dr. Rivera was active in the North Carolina State Medical Association, the National Medical Association and the Allergy Medical Society ("Dr. Tomas Monte Rivera," 1953). When he died in his home on April 14, 1965, his patients were able to go to the recently integrated Wayne County Memorial Hospital for care.

Greenville, Pitt County

St. Frances Hospital, circa 1924–1934

Pitt County, located in the eastern coastal plains region, was originally home to the Tuscarora people. Europeans and enslaved Africans colonized the region in the late 1600s and early 1700s. They drove out, murdered and enslaved the native population. On the eve of the Civil War, in 1860, Pitt County was home to 7,480 white citizens, or about 49 percent of the total population. In addition, there were 8,473 enslaved people and 127 free African Americans for a total African American population of 8,473 or approximately 51 percent of the total population. The populace of Pitt County remained evenly divided between whites and African Americans until out-migration of African Americans after World War II skewed the population to majority white by 1960 (Pitt County, 2016).

When the first hospital in Pitt County, Pitt Community Hospital (PCH), opened in 1924, there were 41 beds for white patients and one bed for an African American patient. Knowing that a single bed was insufficient to meet the needs of African Americans in the region, yet not wanting African Americans to eat or sleep in the hospital, the administrators of PCH paid African American, graduate nurse Frances Hopkins to maintain two beds in her house as the Negro ward of PCH. African Americans had surgery or delivered babies at PCH and then recovered at Nurse Hopkins home/hospital. Nurse Hopkins was a Greenville native with experience in nursing and hospital management. It soon became apparent that three hospital beds did not adequately meet the need for hospital services for over 20,000 African Americans living in Pitt County in 1920 (Williams, 2001).

An article in the local newspaper, the *Daily Reflector*, stated, "everyone has come to realize that a hospital for colored people in Greenville is an immediate and absolute necessity" ("Colored hospital nucleus," 1923, n.p.). To increase the number of hospital beds, Nurse Hopkins leased the Bernard House in downtown Greenville and turned it into the St. Frances Hospital for Colored People (SFHCP). The *Daily Reflector* reported, "The hospital will begin operation on September the first with two graduates and a few class nurses who are making application to the training school" ("Negro hospital to open," 1924). Local civic and church groups made small monthly donations to the new hospital to keep it solvent ("The local Kiwanis," 1924). Pitt County Hospital agreed to allow SFHCP to use its x-ray and sterilizing equipment, operating room and pathology laboratory free of charge. Nurse Hopkins supervised the hospital. Her staff included one other graduate nurse and several nurse's aides. All physicians in the community in good standing were allowed to admit patients at SFHCP. Room, board and nursing care cost $14 a week for women and children less than 12 years of age. Men and older children paid $18 for the same services. Private rooms cost $21 a week regardless of gender or age (Williams, 2001).

In a letter dated September 25, 1924, Nurse Hopkins appealed to the community for donations. She wrote that the SFHCP needed:

> Two more stoves that will burn coal ... 12 blankets, 10 suites of pajamas for men, 17 night dresses for women, 12 pairs of towels, 12 pillow cases, 24 pairs of sheets, 24 counterpanes, curtains for 24 windows.... Second-hand linen will be most acceptable. The St. Frances Hospital for Colored People has at present seven patients. It is depending largely, if not entirely on the Christian charity of the Christian people in the town and county which it is serving [cited in Williams, 2001, p. 30].

In 1934 the administrators of PCH renovated the hospital basement converting it into a 12–15 bed ward for African Americans

(Krammerer, 1986). At that time, the SFHCP closed, and Nurse Hopkins moved to Philadelphia (Williams, 2001).

In 1951 the new Pitt County Memorial Hospital (PCHM) opened its doors and included a 30-bed segregated ward for African American patients on the first floor. In a 1997 oral history, Dr. Andrew Best, a Pitt County African American obstetrician and gynecologist, remembered this ward:

> From the time I came in 1954 for about the following ten years, all the black patients were admitted to the first floor of the east wing ... whether you had pneumonia or a newborn baby you were on the so called colored ward [as cited in Thomas, 1977, p. 82].

The white entrance to the hospital was "located on the front of the building where it was convenient to drive up and walk in" while the African American entrance was in the back of the hospital up a flight of stairs. Threatened with the loss of federal Medicare and Medicaid funding, PCMH finally integrated its beds and staff on May 24, 1965.

Statesville, Iredell County

Colored Branch of Davis Hospital, circa 1925–1940

Pitt Community Hospital was not unique in allowing African American patients in the hospital's operating room, as long as they ate, slept and recovered somewhere else after surgery. Davis Hospital, in Statesville, the county seat of Iredell County, used the same policy.

Iredell County, in the western piedmont section of North Carolina, was originally home to the Cherokee and Catawba people. These Native Americans were displaced in the 1750s by German and Scots-Irish immigrants and enslaved people of African descent (Genealogical society, 1980). In 1860, Iredell's population of 15,347 residents included 11,141 white people, 4,177 enslaved people and 29 free African Americans. By 1930, shortly after the Davis Hospital Negro Annex opened, the population had become whiter, with approximately 30,000 of the total population of 38,000 identified as white, and approximately 8,000 identified as African American (Iredell County, 2016).

Iredell County's first hospital was Billingsley Memorial Hospital

(BMH) in Statesville. It was a gift to the town from the Rev. Amos S. Billingsley, a white Presbyterian minister who came to Statesville after the Civil War to educate the area's newly freed African American people. The Reverend Billingsley died in 1897 and left $5,000 in his will for the construction of a hospital in Statesville with the stipulation that care would be provided to people of both races. It opened in 1900. An article in the March 6, 1908, *Statesville Landmark,* the local newspaper, reported that the hospital had four wards for white patients and a single African American ward in the basement of the building. After BMH closed in 1920, white residents of the county had a choice of two local hospitals—Long Sanatorium or Carpenter-Davis Hospital (by 1925 known as Davis Hospital)—for hospital care. No local health care facilities would admit African Americans (Keever, 1974).

While Billingsley Memorial Hospital was offering limited care to African Americans in its basement ward, a local African American physician opened a small, short-lived, hospital where African Americans could be treated in decent facilities by physicians and nurses of their choice. An item appeared in the October 1, 1912, *Charlotte News* that read:

> Statesville is to have a hospital for colored people. Dr. Holiday, the local colored physician and Frances Clark, a trained nurse from Winston, have rented Mr. E.A. Fry's house on Center Street, not far from Dr. Long's Sanatorium and will convert it into a hospital for the people of their race. There are six rooms in the building. All rooms except the operating room are now ready for the reception of patients and the operating room is not being fitted up ["Colored hospital planned," 1912, p. 7].

The only other mention of the hospital is in a 1912 edition of *Statesville Sentinel*, a local newspaper reporting on a patient being treated in the hospital ("Negro loses foot," 1912).

Around 1925, Davis Hospital officials began allowing white physicians to operate on African Americans patients in the hospital's operating room. From that time until the mid–1940s, African Americans who underwent operations at Davis Hospital were discharged to the home of African American Nurse Daisy Connor Robinson, at 249 Garfield Street, for care (Reese, 2014). Mrs. Robinson also cared for non-surgical patients. An item in the *Statesville Landmark* from 1931 details one such case.

> A Negro man who had been hurt was taken to the Davis hospital and given a free examination by the doctor of the hospital. He was then placed at the

colored hospital on Garfield Street and kept there for fourteen days, at the expense of his board being defrayed jointly by the Associated Charities and the welfare department ["Nurses October report," 1931, p. 5].

Statesville City Directories in the 1930s and 1940s listed "Davis Hospital—Colored Annex" at 249 Garfield Street, Robinson's home address. On April 8, 1932, *The Statesville Landmark* lists Nurse Robinson as receiving $25 from the county for nursing care of indigent patients ("County bills," 1932). Nurse Robinson died of tuberculosis, most likely contracted from a patient, and died in January 1947 at age 54. Robinson's obituary in the January 9th, 1947, *Statesville Landmark* confirms she was in charge of the African American ward at Davis Hospital for a number of years ("Funeral Thursday," 1947, p. 16). She was buried in the African American cemetery in Statesville, and today, no headstone marks her resting place. There are no studies identifying how many other North Carolina hospitals engaged African American nurses as their off-site "colored wards."

Laurinburg, Scotland County

Bigelow Hospital, circa 1926–1949

Scotland County, one of the last counties formed in North Carolina (in 1899), was originally settled by the Cheraw people. Highland Scots, along with English settlers and enslaved Africans, colonized the region in the early 1700s. The area has always been a rural and agricultural with corn, cotton and tobacco being its primary crops (Meyers, 2000). Although Scotland was not a county at the time of the Civil War, in the counties that later made up Scotland County, African Americans made up between 30 percent and 40 percent of the total population (Ptak, 2010). That percentage has remained steady through the present time.

One of the least known African American hospitals in North Carolina was Bigelow Hospital on the campus of the Laurinburg Institute in Laurinburg, North Carolina. Available records indicate it operated from the mid–1920s until the 1950s. Even the dates of its founding and demise are not well documented. Brief mentions in a few newspapers, a designation on a map and a background image in a 1920s photograph of Laurinburg Institute students are all that is left to tell the story of Bigelow Hospital.

The Laurinburg Normal and Industrial Institute was established in 1904 when African American citizens of Scotland County contacted famed African American educator Booker T. Washington at Tuskegee Institute in Alabama, asking him to send teachers to Scotland County to start a school. Emanuel Montee McDuffie and his wife, Tiny, educators trained at Tuskegee, moved to Laurinburg in response to the request. Within a few weeks they opened Laurinburg Institute. Initially, the school had one teacher, seven students, and assets of 15 cents. Ten years later, in 1914, there were 110 students and 13 teachers (Negroes of Scotland County, 1917). The school continued to grow and prosper. In the mid–1920s the school administrators added Bigelow Hospital to its campus. The hospital served students, faculty and staff of the school, and residents of the surrounding area (Wright, 2006).

The *New York Age*, an influential African American newspaper, published 67 items about Bigelow Hospital between 1926 and 1935. Most of these are reports of the health of patients in the hospital. Dr. Nathaniel Edward Jackson, a 1907 graduate of Leonard Medical School, was the founding physician and Nurse A. Elizabeth Patterson was the first nurse. Other physicians who worked at Bigelow Hospital included Dr. Joseph Robinson of Hamlet and a Dr. Hunter ("Laurinburg, NC," 1927). The first mention of Bigelow appeared in the November 20, 1926, edition of the *New York Age* reporting a successful operation ("Laurinburg, NC," 1926). An interesting item in the February 19, 1927, issue of the same paper reported that the Ladies Art Club of Laurinburg gave a shower for Bigelow Hospital, and sheets, pillow cases, bed spreads, towels, and "other appropriate articles" were donated ("Laurinburg, NC," 1927, p. 9). Nurse Patterson resigned in 1928 and was replaced by Geneva H. Culpepper ("Laurinburg, NC," 1928). By 1931, Sadie Alston was Head Nurse ("Laurinburg, NC," 1931). Nurse Alston left after her marriage and was replaced by Bertha McNeil from New York City ("Laurinburg, North Carolina," 1935). An item in the March 30, 1929, *New York Age* mentions that Isabelle DuPree was a student nurse at Bigelow ("Laurinburg, NC," 1929).

Most of the *New York Age* reports detailed patient care at the hospital including the nature of the illness and type of surgery performed. The reports stop in 1935. However, in the April 1949 issue of *The Eastern Searchlight*, a newspaper published by Laurinburg Institute, an advertisement for the Laurinburg Institute includes Bigelow

Hospital as an asset of the school ("The Laurinburg Institute," 1949). There are no other mentions of the hospital in other editions of *The Eastern Searchlight,* and no other information about the hospital is available. For over 20 years, Bigelow Hospital and its staff served the students, teachers and employees at Laurinburg Institute as well as African Americans living in the surrounding area. Perhaps future historians will be able to uncover more of its rich history.

New Bern, Craven County

Good Shepherd Hospital, 1939–1965

The original residents of Craven County, located in the far eastern, central, coastal section of North Carolina, were the Coree and Tuscarora people. As Europeans and enslaved people from Africa settled the land between the Albemarle and Cape Fear Rivers in the decades around 1700, the native population was driven out by war and disease. Craven County's largest city, New Bern, became the county seat in 1722. It was also the capital of colonial North Carolina and first state capital until 1794 (Watson, 1987). The 1860 census shows a majority African American population of 9,190 enslaved people and 1,286 free people, along with a white population of 8,795 (Ptak, 2010). By 1939, when Good Shepherd Hospital opened, about 45 percent of the total population or approximately 14,000 African Americans lived in Craven County (Craven County, 2016). Before GSH was founded the closest modern African American hospitals were in Wilmington, about 100 miles south or Raleigh, about 114 miles east.

Carven County had both more and earlier hospitals than most counties in North Carolina. During the Civil War it was home to two Union hospitals; both the New Bern Academy and the Presbyterian Church were converted into hospitals by Union Troops. In the late 1860s, a Freedmen's Bureau hospital was located there (Watson, 1987). Several hospitals served the white citizens of the county in the early years of the 20th century. Stewart Sanatorium, with 30 beds, was the first modern health care facility in New Bern when it opened on July 15, 1908. Fairview Hospital, frequently referred to as Caton Hospital, opened in 1916. The hospital offered a nurses training program to white women in the 1910s and 1920s. The New Bern General Hospital incorporated as a private hospital on February 25, 1918, with 21 beds and an operating room. St. Luke's Hospital and the St. Luke's Hospital Training School for Nurses was established by physicians J.E. Patterson and R. DuVal Jones in 1929. The Sisters of St. Joseph's of Newark, N.J., bought the hospital in 1944 and operated it until it was bought by the county in 1962. Sadly, none of these hospitals would accept African American patients nor train African American nurses ("Several hospitals," 2013).

A great tragedy occurred in New Bern on December 1, 1922. On that day, a horrendous fire destroyed approximately 40 blocks of African American houses and businesses, leaving thousands of people injured, homeless and unemployed. The fire was of such magnitude

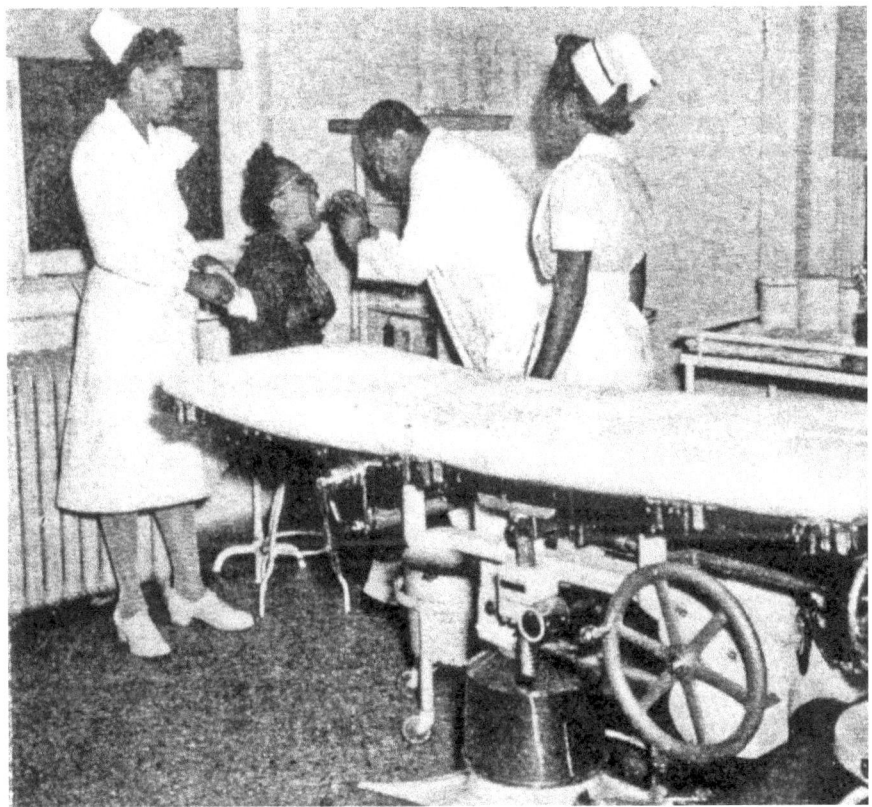

Physicians and nurses providing emergency care, Good Shepherd Hospital, New Bern, 1946 (courtesy Episcopal Diocese of East Carolina).

that state and national officials, the Red Cross and troops stationed at the nearby U.S. Army base at Fort Bragg provided assistance. No local hospitals would accept African American victims of the blaze, so the African American St. Cyprian Episcopal church served as an emergency hospital. The need for a local African American hospital was apparent (Pollitt, 2015).

Bishop Robert C. Darst, and the Rev. Robert I. Johnson of St. Cyprian's Church led the movement to establish a hospital. A local committee of prominent people set out to raise funds, find a suitable site and create community support for the project. The committee envisioned a $200,000, large modern hospital. After an enthusiastic start, including a pledge of $25,000 from the Episcopal Diocese of Pennsylvania, the years of the Great Depression caused delays and setbacks. In 1936, after no other large donations were forthcoming, the Pennsylvania Diocese agreed that their money could be used to construct a small, cottage-style, hospital on land left to the Diocese by the Rev. E.M. Forbes some decades earlier. When officials from the Duke Endowment and the Rosenwald Fund became aware of this plan, they donated $20,000 towards the construction of the Good Shepherd Hospital ("Corner stone," 1938; Embree & Waxman, 1949). Local citizens of both races made small donations to purchase equipment and supplies ("Good Shepherd," 1938).

The hospital opened to great fanfare on June 26, 1938. Speeches were made by Mayor W.C. Chadwick, the Rev. Doctor Charles Screiner from the Diocese of Pennsylvania, Edith Anderson, the White nursing supervisor for Good Shepherd, Graham Davis of the Duke Endowment, Bishop Darst, the Reverend Johnson and others. Hundreds of people witnessed the laying of a cornerstone and enjoyed the singing of the St. Cyprian Church choir. The hospital was an attractive one-story brick structure with three private rooms, 30 ward beds, a nursery, an operating room, an emergency department and outpatient clinic rooms ("Bishop Darst," 1938).

Records for the first full year of operation, July 1, 1938–June 30, 1939, show people from Craven, Carteret, Beaufort, Pamlico, Jones, Onslow, Hyde, Pitt and Lenoir counties utilized hospital services. More than 4,000 people were treated at various out-patient clinics run jointly by the hospital and the county health department including those clinics for tuberculosis, maternity and venereal disease. Eighty cases of "people shot and cut or otherwise battered up" were seen in the Emergency Room that year (Johnson, 1940, p. 1). Almost 700 people were admitted to the hospital for medical care or surgery. The hospital provided 1,164 days of free care at a cost of $3.42 a day (Johnson, 1940). The Duke Endowment donated $1.00 a day towards indigent care, with the rest was covered by local donations from White and African American supporters of the GSH as well as donations from Episcopal groups from around the country. Many members of the local African American community donated fresh and canned food as well as household items and money on "Hospital Day" (Johnson, 1939). In the 1940s all the churches in the Eastern Diocese of the Episcopal Church designated one Sunday a year as "Good Shepherd Hospital Day" with special collections taken up to support the hospital. Good Shepherd celebrated "Hospital Day" each year. The public was invited to classes on many subjects including the human body, personal hygiene and home nursing of the sick (Report to the community, 1948).

Both African American and White physicians admitted and cared for patients in the hospital. African American physicians included Drs. Mumford, Mann, Fisher and Martin; White physicians using the Good Shepherd Hospital in the 1940s included Drs. Duffey, Wadsworth, Ashford and Kafer. In 1939, Miss Rebecca Hennie succeeded Miss Anderson and nursing supervisor (Johnson, 1940).

Throughout the 1940s and 1950s, the hospital and the number of patients grew. GSH received an "A" rating from the American Hospital and American Medical Associations and the American College of Surgeons and was licensed by the North Carolina Medical Care Commission (Ryan, 1964). Both Craven County and the city of New Bern made annual contributions as did various Episcopal organizations. In 1944 the federal government paid for a 25-bed addition to the hospital as well as a new Nurse's Home. The 10th anniversary "Report to the community" published in 1948 gives statistics for 1947. In that year 825 patients received 7,441 days of care, 296 operations were performed and 122 babies were delivered. By 1953 the number of inpatients had increased to 1,236, the number of outpatient visits to 1,106 and 391 operations were performed. The nursing staff had doubled to eight graduate nurses. The 17 other hospital employees included orderlies, nurse's aides, housekeepers, dietary staff, a laboratory and x-ray technician, the hospital administrator and a secretary (Report to the community, 1948). Nurses who worked at Good Shepherd Hospital

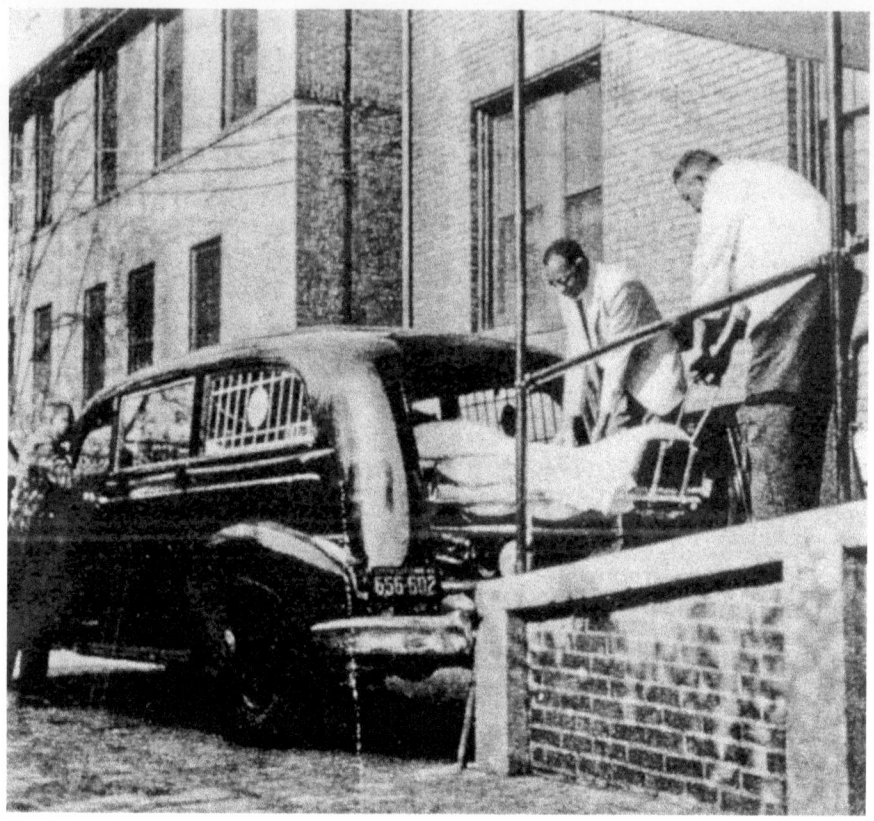

Patients discharged at Good Shepherd Hospital, New Bern, 1946 (courtesy Episcopal Diocese of East Carolina).

included Miss Rebecca Hennie, Miss M.L. Phillips, Mrs. V.C. Davis, Mrs. M. H. Skinner, Laura Moore, Doris Adams, Inez Dudley Frances, Parnelle Shaw and Marchusa Armstrong (Johnson, 1941; Johnson, 1950).

Two major changes to the hospital occurred in 1954. First, Dr. Lula Dissoway, a native white New Bernian physician, became the Medical Director of the Hospital and served in that capacity until the hospital closed in 1967. Dr. Dissoway had spent the prior decades as an Episcopal medical missionary to China and Alaska but returned home to care for her ailing mother. At Good Shepherd Hospital and later at Craven County Hospital she organized free prenatal clinics, delivered babies and taught classes in child care for new parents in the local community (Mega, Mega, & King, 2000). Secondly, another new wing, costing $90,000 was added. Three years later a hospital chapel was completed (London & Lemmon, 1987). A 1964 newspaper article described Good Shepherd Hospital.

> Good taste and attractiveness seem to be part of Good Shepherd's system of therapy. The rooms, larger than most found in present-day hospitals, are nicely furnished and attractively painted. This goes, too, for hallways, offices, lounges, staff dining rooms and the kitchen [Ryan, 1964, p. 5].

In 1964, responding to the *Simkins v. Moses Cone* court decision and the Civil Rights Act of 1964, Craven County took over the management and ownership of Good Shepherd Hospital from the Episcopal Diocese of East Carolina. The county integrated the formerly white-only Craven County Hospital and replaced the formerly all-white Hospital Board with two African Americans and three whites (Tan seats, 1965). Good Shepherd operated as an integrated hospital until 1966 when it became a nursing home and continues to serve the community in that capacity today.

Tarboro, Edgecombe County

Quigless Clinic, 1946–1974

For hundreds of years, the Tuscarora people lived in the area that became Edgecombe County, in the eastern piedmont region. As Europeans and enslaved Africans moved onto Tuscarora lands in the late 1600s and early 1700s, conflict ensued. The Tuscarora people were devastated by new diseases and lost armed battles against the settlers in what are known as the Tuscarora Wars of 1711–1715. Most Native American survivors moved north to live with related tribes. The European and African American population grew and the new residents created many large plantations growing tobacco, cotton, wheat and corn. In 1860, at the beginning of the Civil War, Edgecombe County's population was 58 percent African American and 42 percent white (Srikanth, 2016). This ratio stayed virtually unchanged for 150 years. The 2010 U.S. Census reveals that the population of Edgecombe County was approximately 57 percent African American, almost 40 percent white and 3 percent other races.

Despite being a majority African American county for a century and a half, two of the earliest hospitals in the county, Pittman Hospital (1901–1916) and Bass Memorial Hospital (1929–1959), were white-only institutions, and Edgecombe General Hospital (1916–1959) added a small "Colored Annex" in 1920. African American physicians were banned from practicing in all of these hospitals (Watson, 1979). Dr. Milton Douglas Quigless was one of those banned physicians. He recalled one of his early experiences in Edgecombe County:

> Most people didn't have any damn money.... They were all sharecroppers and what not. I remember this lady. She was in labor and her husband ran in one day. Said, "Doc, come out right quick and see about my wife." She lived about ten miles out in the country. So I went out there. The lady had had a precipitous labor. That the baby just burst out every damn thing. Lacerated the vagina, lower part of the intestines, the uterus. Every damn thing and blood was just shooting out. Put a sheet up there. Told my receptionist to come out with some ether. She poured the damn ether and I had to sew on that lady about an hour and a half. Well, she healed all right except for one little place. And we got along very well. No blood transfusion. Hell, wasn't no blood bank or nothing in those days. The Lord just wasn't ready for her to go [Chafe, Gavins & Korstad, 2001, p. 24].

He recounted a visit to a local dentist's office:

> I went to his office and saw he had one waiting room for whites and a different one for blacks. He had an operating room for whites with up-to-date equipment. He also had an operating room for blacks, the same room in which the brooms and mops were kept along with equipment that wasn't in such good condition [Quigless, 1994, p.138].

Milton Douglas Quigless was born in Port Gibson, Mississippi on August 16, 1904, to John and Agnes Quigless. He graduated from Meharry Medical College (MMC) in Nashville in 1934 and then completed an internship at the Homer G. Phillips Hospital in St. Louis. Dr. Quigless returned to MMC and taught physiology for a year before arriving in Tarboro, with seven dollars in his pocket, to begin a clinical practice. He chose Tarboro because the area had not had an African American physician for several years prior to his arrival. Shortly after his arrival in 1936, Tarboro city officials gave Dr. Quigless six months of free rent to establish his new clinic in an abandoned fish market on Main Street, next to the Tar River (Quigless, 1994). He remembers the dismal state of health care for African Americans in Edgecombe County before he built the Quigless Clinic-Hospital.

> I was here ten years and I couldn't get into the hospital. Black people were dying in the country. I had to go out to the sharecropper shacks and operate on

people with the light from a flashlight. One white man told me "You're not a doctor, you're a black bastard." I used to carry a gun when I went out to the shacks. I got fed up with it and I decided to start my own hospital [Fleishman, 1994, p. 1].

Dr. Quigless had been in Tarboro about four years when the United States entered World War II. Several local white physicians joined the armed services and left Tarboro to serve. Their absence was the catalyst for Dr. Quigless to be offered a job managing the health department during the war years. In his autobiography, *Looking back: The way things were*, Dr. Quigless describes the events that precipitated his opening of his hospital.

> One night I got a call from a family living about eight miles from Tarboro. I went out to find that the lady had been in labor for three days. It was quite evident that the baby was dead. The mother's pains had ceased completely and she was developing symptoms of infection. The family had no money, and even if they had, I doubt that I could have gotten her into a hospital anywhere in the vicinity. So it was up to me to do whatever I could to save her life. I went back to Tarboro, picked up my receptionist and a couple of cans of ether.... It was July and hot. There were no screens on the window ... after the administration of the ether I started pulling out the fetus. I pulled and tugged for over two hours. As I was doing this, the flies were crawling all over my face and I wasn't able to brush them off.... On the way back to town, I said "Mrs. Beamon, I'm going to have to build that damn hospital right away. I can't stand much more of this." I'm glad you said that because I can't stand much more either" she agreed [1994, p. 150].

In December 1946, Dr. Quigless opened the Quigless Clinic-Hospital, the first hospital in Edgecombe County built to serve African Americans. The original 25-bed hospital had a reception room, outpatient clinic, ward and nurse's quarters on the first floor. Women's and pediatric wards as well as the delivery room and operating room were on the second floor. The Clinic-Hospital also included an x-ray room, kitchen, dining room, storage room and laboratory. Dr. Quigless's wife Helen ran the business office, dietary department, human resources, maintenance department, and she sewed the curtains. Dr. Quigless bought many used items to equip his hospital including an operating table salvaged from a World War II battleship. His initial staff included another physician, three graduate nurses, one of whom was a registered nurse who graduated from Good Samaritan Hospital in Charlotte, two local high school girls who worked as nursing assistants, a cook and an orderly (Quigless, 1994). In order to provide the highest quality care, Dr. Quigless frequently consulted with specialists around the state. In the days before penicillin he improvised and occasionally used folk and herbal remedies to help his patients (Reed, 2008).

An article in the February 27, 1996, *Daily Southerner* describes the early days of the hospital:

> Ironically, some of the doctor's first patients were white, "Believe it or not (blacks) were the very folks who wouldn't come see me once I got here" Quigless said. "At first (whites) only came late at night (for fear of being seen visiting the black doctor), but that was all right. Some of them came because they heard I was a good doctor. Back then I didn't ask questions; I was thankful to have some paying customers." Some customers paid with money; others helped the doctor furnish his office; some paid with chicken, eggs –whatever they could [Harris, p. 8].

Dr. Milton Quigless, Jr., remembered his father's work this way:

> One day he was taking out an appendix, the next he was performing a hysterectomy and putting someone in traction and taking and interpreting his own x-rays—then going out and delivering a baby ["Doctor," 1994, p. 7].

Dr. Quigless and his Clinic-Hospital served the African American community in and around Tarboro through the civil rights era. In 1973, North Carolina Medical Commission representatives surveyed the Quigless Clinic and found that it did not meet the current building codes for hospitals. The renovations necessary to meet the building codes were prohibitively expensive. At that time, Dr. Quigless closed the hospital portion of his facility but kept his office and clinic open (Quigless, 1994). By then, the Edgecombe General Hospital was fully integrated, and Dr. Quigless was on the hospital staff. Dr. Quigless continued seeing patients well into his 80s. He delivered over 3,000 babies, many named after him (both his first and middle names: Milton and Douglas) and his wife, Helen. By the 1990s, Dr. Quigless received many honors and awards for his courageous work and wrote his autobiography (Dudley, 1987; Doles, 1987). Dr. Quigless died in Tarboro on November 18, 1997 (Reed, 2008).

Fayetteville, Cumberland County

Leary-Perry Hospital, 1950–1955

For over 10,000 years, various Souian tribes including the Eno, Shakori, Waccamaw, and Keyauwee inhabited the land that became

Cumberland County in southeastern North Carolina. By the 1720s, Highland Scots, other Europeans and enslaved Africans began moving into the area. On the eve of the Civil War, in 1860, out of Cumberland County's 16,369 residents, there were 9,561 whites, 6,830 enslaved people and 978 free African Americans (Ptak, 2010). In the first half of the 20th century, many African Americans had migrated north in search of employment and a better life in states without segregation. By 1950, the percentage of African Americans in the county had dropped from almost 50 percent in 1860 to 30 percent by 1950 (Cumberland County, 2016).

In 1901, Dr. Jacob Franklin Highsmith of Fayetteville, the county seat of Cumberland County, established Highsmith Hospital as the first private hospital in North Carolina. With the help of Dr. William Thomas Rainey, the hospital grew into one of the leading medical facilities in the region. At Highsmith Hospital, regardless of diagnosis, all African Americans were placed together in a single basement ward. Space was a problem, and African Americans were turned away if the basement ward was full, even if there were many empty beds upstairs (Clement, 2001). Residents in the counties around Fayetteville were designated as one of three primary racial groups: Whites, African Americans and Lumbee Indians. Racial laws and customs reflected the varying status of each of these groups. When African American physician Dr. C. Mason Quick was asked about the differences in facilities for each race inside Highsmith Hospital, he responded:

> [The differences] were night and day. But they [hospital administrators] also had a problem with the Indians [primarily Lumbee Indians], if they [Lumbees] didn't want to be with us. The [hospital administrators] didn't want them with whites, so they had a little section they would put the Indians if they objected to being with the Negroes [McQueen, 2014, p. 1].

African American physicians were allowed to treat their patients in the basement ward, but could not treat hospitalized white patients nor join the Fayetteville chapter of the all-white North Carolina Medical Society (McQueen, 2014).

In August of 1917, Dr. Chester Arthur Eaton, a Henderson native and 1910 graduate of Leonard Medical School, opened his first office in Lumberton in 1910 ("This week in Lumberton," 1910; Caldwell, 1921). Within a few years, he founded a sanitorium to treat African Americans on Hillsboro Street in Fayetteville. At that time, the tax-supported North Carolina State Sanitarium, located in neighboring Hoke County, was 10 years old, but refused to accept African American patients. A short piece in the August 22, 1917, *Fayetteville Weekly Observer* noted:

> Dr. C.A. Eaton, one of the leading colored physicians, has established in what was formerly the McQueen hotel Hillsboro Street, a sanitorium for the colored people. This is a move in the right direction, and there is no reason it should not be successful, as an institution of the kind is needed here [p. 1].

For reasons that have not been recorded, Dr. Eaton's Sanatorium did not last long. Shortly after leaving Fayetteville, Dr. Eaton moved to Winston-Salem and maintained a thriving private practice for many years (Ancestry.com, 2016). Once again the colored basement ward of Highsmith Hospital was the only locally available health care facility that accepted African American patients. Until 1942, African Americans living in Cumberland County who wanted to be treated by doctors and nurses of their own race traveled at least 50 miles to reach any of the African American hospitals in existence at that time.

Dr. Mathew Leary Perry had the vision and the determination to change the situation. Dr. Perry was born in Fayetteville in 1892 to Dallas and Mary Leary Perry. He attended local schools before graduating from Fayetteville State Normal School and earning his medical degree at Leonard Medical School in 1908. Perry opened his first office in Maxton. In World War I he was a commissioned First Lieutenant in the Officers Reserve Corps. Dr. Perry joined Dr. N.E. Jackson to staff the Bigelow Hospital at the Laurinburg Institute in the 1920s, and with his brother, Dr. John S. Perry, opened the Mercy Hospital in Hamlet, about 50 miles away, around the same time (Womble, 2002). In October 1932, during the Great Depression, the Perry brothers opened the Provident Health Center at 613 Nun Street serving indigent people in Wilmington. Their practice focused on people with tuberculosis, heart disease and venereal diseases. By 1940, Dr. Perry had opened a private practice in Fayetteville (Oates, 1950).

In 1941, at the outbreak of World War II, he led a unique experiment in nursing education. Fayetteville is home to Fort Bragg, one of the largest U.S. Army bases in the United States. Fort Bragg was founded in 1918, and the first permanent base hospital was erected in 1932. In 1940, with the expectation that the U.S. would soon be entering World War II, the population at Fort Bragg expanded from 5,400 to 67,000 (Fort Bragg, 2013). Seeing an opportunity for employment for local African American women, Dr. Mathew Leary Perry opened a school of practical nursing. An article in the *Fayetteville Observer* informed its readers about this unique endeavor:

> A colored nursing school, said to be one of the first to be established in the south, will open its doors for classes on January 4 ... to make it possible for young colored women to equip themselves for a work greatly in demand. The course of instruction will follow modern teaching and include classroom and laboratory work, sickroom experiences and bedside practice. Visual instruction will be presented in the form of moving pictures to illustrate important facts concerning disease and care of the sick ... some 14 colored women from five eastern counties have already signed up for the course which will extend over 18 months. Certifications will be awarded students upon completion of the course ["Colored nursing school," 1941, p. 2].

The article further explained that an infirmary, open to local residents, had already been set up at 115 1/2 Gillespie Street, and an accompanying out-patient clinic would open at the same location. These facilities would provide care for local people and at the same time be the primary clinical site for the students to learn their nursing skills ("Colored nursing school," 1941). Officials at Fort Bragg allowed six of their nurses to become instructors at the school and hired many of the school's graduates. Oates (1950) notes, "A large number of women completed the course and entered the field of nurses-aids" (p. 246).

After the war years, Dr. Perry turned his attention to opening a hospital for women and children. His dream was realized on June 6th, 1950, when he opened the Leary-Perry Hospital for Women and Newborns at 334 Moore St. in Fayetteville. Dr. Perry explained the need for his new hospital:

> Statistics point out that expectant mothers, even where complications exist, often find it impossible to be admitted to general hospitals or to secure the services of a physician ... our southern states report that 83% of all colored births are attended by unschooled midwives ["Maternity home," 1949, n.p.].

A front page article titled *Negro maternity hospital hailed as major help in medical care* in the June 19th, 1950 edition of *The Fayetteville Observer* gave a detailed account of the facility. The building was 6,000 square feet with a reception area, two examination rooms, two delivery rooms, one operating room, a sterilizing room, a laboratory, a physical therapy room, a fully equipped kitchen, sleeping rooms for physicians, two nurse's stations, 40 patient beds, composed of semi-private rooms, wards and bassinets. There were florescent lights, hot and cold running water, steam-heat and water fountains. Two other buildings were on the hospital grounds. One housed a nurse's dormitory, business offices, a medical records room and an out-patient clinic; the other was a laundry house. The hospital complex was completed for a total cost of $23,000 with the Fort Bragg Community Chest being the largest benefactor, contributing $8,000 to equip the hospital with needed supplies. The first nurses were Mrs. Henry L. Wooten and Mrs. O.H. Lincoln. Although the hospital treated only obstetrical and pediatric cases, it provided more care to African Americans by African American physicians than had ever been available in Fayetteville.

In the first two months of operation, the hospital admitted 50 patients and 19 births were recorded ("New center here," 1950). However, the hospital quickly faced financial problems. An article in *The Fayetteville Observer* published only two months after the hospital's opening noted:

> Fayetteville's recently opened Negro maternity hospital is in urgent need of funds ... although much equipment is still needed, most of the money being requested at this time is for current operating costs. If funds are not raised, continued operation of the hospital will be impossible ["Colored maternity hospital," 1950, p. 2].

By the end of August 1950, local individuals, service clubs and businesses had contributed over $500 to the hospital. Unfortunately, these donations were not enough to keep the hospital open in the days before private health insurance, Medicare, Medicaid and the Affordable Care Act. The date of the hospital's closure has not been recorded, but the hospital has been described as short lived ("Exchange Club," 1950; Womble, 2002). It took 13 years after Dr. Perry's hospital closed for Cape Fear Valley Hospital, a public, tax-supported institution, to fully integrate its admission and staffing policies. The private Highsmith Memorial Hospital followed three months later, integrating its facility on November 15, 1963 (Jacobs, 2013).

Conclusion

These brief sketches of 39 health care institutions founded by and/or for African Americans during the Jim Crow era in North Carolina are but glimpses into the complete and complex histories of each institution. Additional scholarship will reveal more about the people, the communities and the political, economic, religious and social influences that shaped each one. In addition to learning more about the institutions presented in this book, illusive mentions of several other African American hospitals in many North Carolina cities are found in newspaper articles and other sources. For instance, the founding of an African American hospital in High Point is noted in an article in *The High Point Enterprise* on October 1, 1912:

> The colored hospital which has been improvised to take care of those needing medical and surgical treatment is doing a good work. It is situated on the Moon property east of the Colored Normal school. It is under the auspices of the colored physicians here ["Colored hospital," 1912, p. 1].

Two years later, another article titled "Negro Slashed with Razor-Wounds Serious" on the front page of the February 9, 1914, *The High Point Enterprise* reads in part: "The wounded Negro is at the colored hospital here, and it is probable that his wound will prove fatal." Similarly, the first mention of an African American hospital in Wadesboro appeared in the November, 20, 1917, *The Messenger Intelligencer* of Wadesboro. Columnist Mrs. J.G. Boylin opined: "We need a colored hospital. The boys are going to the front [World War I] and they are going to need attention. All of our darkies have to go to Charlotte for treatment" ("Women's and children's division," 1922, p. 6). Three years later another article informed its readers on the front page of the January 29, 1920, edition that Mr. R.E. Little made a donation to erect an African American hospital in Wadesboro. The hospital plans included six private rooms, two eight-bed wards and an operating room. The article concluded, "The colored hospital would fill a long felt want here. At present a colored person needing hospital treatment must go to Charlotte or further" ("New hospital facilities," 1920, p. 1). Another item in *The Messenger Intelligencer* dated November, 16, 1922, stated: "Mae Henry, one of the graduate nurses who has been at the colored hospital since it opened more than a year ago, left last week for a rest. Geogiana Burch, a nurse from Good Samaritan Hospital in Charlotte will take her place" ("Anson Sanitarium News," 1922, p. 1). Apparently, Shelby was also home to a short-lived and unstudied hospital. An item in *The Cleveland Star* announced, "The colored hospital is open and ready to receive patients" on the seventh page of its November 2, 1923, edition. More recently, Womble (2002) notes, "The brothers [physicians John S. Perry and Mathew Perry] also owned and operated Mercy Hospital in Hamlet for a number of years" (n.p.). Parker (1990) wrote in his *Cumberland County: A Brief History* that Highsmith Hospital, the leading white hospital in Fayetteville, did not admit African American patients until 1965. However: "Mrs. Cochran, a New York heiress, bought a residence next door to the facility [Highsmith Hospital] had it refurbished as the 'Cochran Wing' and designated it for use by black and indigent sufferers" (p. 96). Details about these and possibly other African American hospitals in the state remain obscure. Future scholars may be able to flesh out their stories. A deeper understanding of the forces that supported as well as those that hindered the success of each hospital, clinic and sanatorium will help guide policy makers today and in the future as they grapple with the ongoing interplay between race, health and public institutions.

Although the days of legal segregation have been over for more than half a century, lingering effects of slavery, segregation and racism continue to affect the health of many North Carolinians today. The Center for Disease Control report on minority health in 2014 mirrored similar findings from the early 1900s:

> Health disparities between African Americans and other racial and ethnic populations are striking and apparent in life expectancy, death rates, infant mortality, and other measures of health status and risk conditions and behaviors [Black or African American, n.d., p. 1].

Eliminating health disparities based on race will require constant vigilance and action by health care policy makers and providers. The Center for Disease Control asserts that:

> Achieving health equity requires valuing everyone equally with focused and ongoing societal efforts to address avoidable inequalities, historical and contemporary injustices, and the elimination of health and healthcare disparities.[Disparities, n.d., p. 1].

This book seeks to fill a void by addressing historical injustices in hospital care for African Americans in North Carolina. As hospitals were established around the turn of the 20th century, most African American patients were not admitted to segregated white hospitals, or would languish in sub-standard Colored wards if they were allowed inside at all. Only through the establishment and maintenance of African American hospitals and public health efforts did life expectancy and the state of health improve for many African Americans. Their most important contributions were addressing the health needs of African American people, providing training and employment for African American health care professionals and being battlegrounds in the struggle for Civil Rights. African American hospitals, some established by churches and supported by white benefactors, the majority founded by African American physicians, provided hundreds of thousands of days of care, many to indigent patients. Not all of these hospitals were successful or long lived, but they demonstrated the courage and tenacity of physicians, nurses and communities to meet their own health needs under dire circumstances.

In addition to fulfilling their primary function of providing care to the ill, injured and dying, African American hospitals were points of pride in their communities. In the darkest days of racial apartheid, with restrictive laws and policies diminishing every aspect of life for African Americans in North Carolina, the very existence of these professional institutions—managed by, funded by and supporting—African American communities, gave lie to the myth of African American inferiority.

In the 50-plus years since the Fourth Circuit Court of Appeals ruling in *Simkins v. Moses H. Cone Memorial Hospital* in 1963, the passage of the Civil Rights Act of 1964 and the implementation of Medicare and Medicaid in 1965, racial bias has decreased markedly in health care. There are no longer separate hospital wards designated by race nor do white physicians routinely refuse to treat African American patients. African American health care providers have been employed in every hospital in North Carolina and are accepted into every public and private medical, nursing, dental and pharmacy school in the state. While health disparities between the races continue, trying to eliminate them has become a national priority. While history can teach us all where we came from and give us guidance for the future, it is also history that teaches us to hope. As Confederate General Robert E. Lee reflected after the Civil War:

> The march of Providence is so slow and our desires so impatient; the work of progress so immense and our means of aiding it so feeble; the life of humanity is so long, that of the individual so brief, that we often see only the ebb of the advancing wave and are thus discouraged. It is history that teaches us to hope.

Appendix I
Publicly Supported Specialty Hospitals for African Americans in North Carolina

While this book focuses on private, church-related and other non-tax supported African American hospitals, this short section briefly addresses the three state-funded African American hospitals in North Carolina. They differed from the other hospitals described in this book in significant ways. First, because they were established and maintained with tax money, they did not face the financial hardships that often devastated the private and non-profit hospitals. The Negro divisions of the state-supported tuberculosis sanitarium and orthopedic hospital remained open until they were no longer needed. The psychiatric hospital in Goldsboro still operates as an integrated institution. Secondly, most of the top administrators were white while all the patients and most of the staff were African Americans. The policies, pay rates and other administrative decisions were made by officials in Raleigh. These hospitals did not involve the local community as members on decision making committees nor did they seek funds from the communities in which they were established. Instead of answering a need in a local community, these state-funded hospitals opened to comply with the U.S. Supreme Court *Plessy v. Ferguson* decision mandating "separate but equal" public facilities. They were formed later than and had fewer staff and services than their white counterparts. These hospitals did provide needed care for many African Americans suffering from various maladies, and the nursing school associated with the Negro Division of the State Sanitarium educated over 100 young women into the nursing profession.

After the Civil War, when Union troops controlled the former Confederate states, national laws and policies promising equal access to public institutions were enforced throughout the south. In the years around the turn of the 20th century, North Carolina governors and legislators chose to enact segregation laws and create racially segregated state institutions. To comply with the 1896 *Plessy v. Ferguson* U.S. Supreme Court decision, institutions were allowed to be segregated by race, but were supposed to be of equal quality. State tax monies were used to establish and maintain three different sets of "separate but equal" specialty hospitals. Not only did the hospitals skirt federal law by underfunding and staffing of the African American institutions, so they were in no way equal to the white institution, but also this system of segregation wasted public funds by duplicating administrative, educational and clinical services. The three specialty hospitals for African Americans were the Asylum for the Colored Insane in Goldsboro, the Negro Wing of the State Orthopedic Hospital near Gastonia and the Negro Division of the North Carolina [tuberculosis] Sanitarium in Hoke County. These institutions were racially separate, but never equal. African American patients received proportionately fewer funds, less staff, poorer facilities and had higher patient to physician ratios than did their white counterparts.

Goldsboro, Wayne County

The Asylum for the Colored Insane (now Cherry Hospital)

The first segregated state-funded institution was the Asylum for the Colored Insane. As noted in the introduction, Union troops controlled Raleigh and all of North Carolina by the middle of April 1865. On April 13, 1865, within days of the Confederate surrender, the Union Provost Marshall in Raleigh ordered the first African American patient, a Union soldier, be admitted to Dix Hospital (DH), the only state-owned psychiatric hospital located in Raleigh. Local African American residents soon followed. Due to federal Reconstruction era laws ensuring parity for both races in public facilities, Dix Hospital was racially integrated for a decade and a half, until the state began enacting segregation laws. Due to overcrowding at DH and the enactment of apartheid laws in North Carolina, in the 1870s and 1880s, the state erected two additional psychiatric hospitals, one for African Americans in Goldsboro and one for white patients in Morganton (Dorothea Dix Hospital, 2014).

In August 1880, the 76-bed Asylum for the Colored Insane opened with a dozen African American patients who were transferred from DH. By Christmas of that year there were over 100 patients living there (Cherry Hospital, 2016). An item in *The Institutional Care of the Insane in the United States and Canada, Volume 3* described the new hospital:

> Owning to the fact that insanity has increased markedly among the Negro's following their emancipation ... a farm of 170 acres one and a half miles west of the town and on Little River was purchased for $5,000 ... the first buildings were erected on a hill beautifully shaded by massive oaks, 400 yards from the river. They consisted of a four story brick administration building and adjoining

it on the south a three-story brick building 36 by 150 feet for the accommodation of patients [Hurd, 1916, p. 285].

According to the 1880 U.S. Census, there were 450 African Americans in the state classified as "insane." Because no private psychiatric facilities in North Carolina admitted African American patients, at least 350 people identified with mental illness had no appropriate care available to them. In 1884 a new dormitory was erected at CH, increasing the bed capacity to 160 (Superintendent's report, 1884). Disparities in funding between the white and African American state psychiatric hospitals were addressed in the 1904 Superintendent's Annual Report. Superintendent Miller wrote:

> The Negro population, approximately, is one-third of the white population, and yet the state has expended for buildings and other equipments for the care of her colored insane but little more than one-sixth as much as for the care of the white insane [Miller, 1905, p. 7].

The causes of mental illness were poorly understood in the 19th and early 20th centuries. Some of the early admitting diagnoses at CH were religion or religious excitement, epilepsy, domestic trouble, bereavement, heredity, masturbation, blow to the head, uterine trouble and extreme heat. Regardless of diagnosis, all patients were given the same general treatment (Superintendent's report, 1884).

Diagnosis of Patients at Cherry Hospital, 1884

	Males	Females	Totals
Unknown	5	21	26
Religion and religious excitement	4	3	7
Epilepsy	7	1	8
Domestic trouble	2	3	5
Death of wife	2	0	2
Hereditary	0	1	1
Masturbation	1	0	1
Blow on head	0	1	1
Uterine trouble	0	4	4
Sunstroke or extreme heat	1	1	2
Brain disease	1	0	1
Destitution	1	1	2
Jealousy	2	0	2
Superstition	0	2	2
Financial troubles	1	0	1
Grief	0	1	1
Intemperance (drunkenness and excessive drink)	3	0	3
Protracted illness	3	0	3
Disappointment in love	0	1	1
Cerebral Congestion	0	1	1
Puerperal	0	1	1

	Males	Females	Totals
Exposure	1	0	1
Sequelae to typhoid fever	1	0	1
Hard study	0	1	1
Deranged Menses	0	1	1
Paralysis	1	0	1
Syphilis	1	0	1
Total	37	44	81

Source: 1882–1884 Biennial Report.

Cherry Hospital, like Dix and Broughton hospitals for white patients, as well as many other psychiatric hospitals of the time, used the colony treatment method. Hospitals using this method were intended to function as a self-sustaining therapeutic colony or village. The colony buildings and surroundings were created to provide patients with a serene, home-like experience (Grob, 1994). Dr. Frederick Peterson, of New York, in an address before the Medico-Psychological Association explained:

> We do not have an institution after all, not a corridored agglomeration of huge pavilions, not a palatial barrack for hundreds of patients of all classes, but a farming hamlet, a village community, if you please.... Healthful outdoor exercise on the farm has been found to be the best treatment as well as the most remunerative [Shrandy & Stedman, 1899, p. 775].

Female patients participated in "work therapy" in housekeeping, soap making, the laundry, the sewing rooms, the canning rooms, the kitchen gardens and the kitchen. The 1884 Annual Report for the institution reports:

> We continue to work our female patients in the sewing room under Miss Kennedy's direction. Mrs. Smith reports nearly a thousand pieces of clothing made during the year, and 1,700 mended. Fifteen patch work quilts, many of them of unique design, (crazy quilts) made of homespun, have been made during the year [p. 16].

Male patients worked on the institution's farm growing crops and tending livestock that provided most of the food for the patients and staff. The 1884 Annual Report reflects the variety of food stuffs produced at the institution:

> Our farm did hardly as well as usual this year. The Steward reports 80 barrels corn, 6,000 pounds of fodder, 50 bushels of peas gathered, and 3,000 pounds of oats. We now have 37 hogs for butchering and estimate their weight at 4,000 pounds. We lost 75 hogs from the cholera in the Spring. We now have 60 hogs for another year, including sows, shoats and pigs. An accurate account of the vegetables has not been kept, and the value of our kitchen garden can hardly be estimated. The orchard again gave us apples in abundance. The cows bought in the winter have done well through the year. They, with their calves, took several premiums at the Fair of the "Eastern Carolina Fair and Stock Association" in November. One of the cows is disposed to go dry early, and, as she is now

worth as much for beef as her original cost, I shall so use her and purchase another for milk [p. 16].

The men also did construction jobs at the facility. Despite these pleasant-sounding treatment methods, patient mistreatment and abuse occasionally occurred at CH, as it did at many large psychiatric hospitals. According to Thomas (2006), "In 1937, an investigation by ... the Department of Public Welfare uncovered shocking conditions of neglect and use of mental patients as maintenance, child care, and field laborers even after they were eligible for discharge" (p. 843).

Social Worker Vanessa Jackson reports in her training manual *Separate and unequal: The legacy of separate and unequal psychiatric hospital*:

> The Cherry Hospital Museum offer insight into what types of treatment patients would have experienced during certain times. On the side porch stands a wooden replica of a large iron cage in which violent and manic patients would be placed.... Dr. Mintauts Vault was reportedly appalled when he arrived in 1956 to assume the Superintend post and discovered the iron cage. He crusaded for better conditions and treatment of his patients. Dr. Vault discovered that in 1957–58 the state spent $866 dollars per patient at Cherry Hospital while per capita expenditures at the all-white hospitals ranged from $1,477 to $1,844.... African American patients were routinely leased to local white farmers to pick their cotton and other crops. Even if one can accept the therapeutic value of laboring in the fields to produce food for patient consumption, there was absolutely no justification for send African American patients out to perform painful and back-breaking work for local farmers [Jackson, 2001, p. 17].

The hospital grew in both number of patients and staff and the number of buildings at the facility. By 1921 there were 960 patient beds. A separate building was established for treating tubercular patients. In addition, a building for the criminally insane was opened in 1924. By 1938 there were approximately 2,500 patients and 123 physicians at CH (Reports of the State Hospital, 1922, 1924 and 1940). A leading figure in the early years of CH was Dr. William W. Faison, the first African American psychiatrist in North Carolina. He was born on August 16, 1854, as a slave on the Pleasant Retreat Plantation near Turkey, North Carolina. Dr. Faison was educated in local schools and graduated from the Jefferson Medical College in Philadelphia in 1878. He dedicated 43 years of his life and career to the patients at CH. From 1883 to 1906, he served as First Assistant Physician and from 1906 until his death in 1926 as head of the institution (Carter, 1957). A biographical dictionary of physicians from Sampson County noted:

> A distinguished alienist [psychiatrist], he spent forty-three years in trying to improve the condition of the unfortunate Negro insane—he was definitely a pioneer in this field. A colleague says of his work, "A prosaic life but one entirely suited to a man of his mental habits and high ideals of service ... as a

result of his wisdom and industry the Goldsboro Institution holds high rank among its class. He was a friend whom it was an honor to call friend" Carter, 1957, p. 24].

After World War II, with advances in pharmacology and surgery, prior approaches to treating psychiatric disorders were largely replaced by a medical treatment model. In the 1930s, across the country, as well as at CH, lobotomies were introduced and electric shock treatments became common place in the 1940s. Effective new psychiatric medications began to be routinely administered to institutionalized patients; many of whom became able to manage their disorders in community settings (Grob, 1994).

Two important new federal laws passed in the 1960s that had large impacts on CH. The first occurred in 1963. The U.S. Congress passed the Community Mental Health Act (CMHA) which established new community mental health centers. The purpose of the CMHA was to build mental health centers to provide community-based care as an alternative to institutionalization. Patients could be treated at the centers while working and living at home (Grob, 1994). The number of inpatients in Cherry Hospital, as well as Broughton and Dix hospitals was greatly reduced. The second was the passage of the Civil Rights Act of 1964, banning racial segregation in public, tax-supported facilities. For CH's first 85 years, it served the entire African American population of the State of North Carolina. In 1965, when North Carolina began complying with the Civil Rights Act of 1964, CH began serving African American and white patients from the 33 most eastern counties in the state. African American patients at CH who were residents of other counties were transferred to hospitals in their appropriate region (Cherry Hospital, 1997). Soon after integration, many improvements were made at Cherry Hospital. More and better trained staff were hired, maintenance improved and new facilities were added.

Sanatorium, Hoke County

Negro Division of the North Carolina Sanatorium, 1923–1965

The second state-supported African American specialty hospital to open was the Negro Division of the State Sanatorium in Sanatorium (now McCain), North Carolina. In the late 19th and early 20th century, tuberculosis was a leading cause of death in North Carolina and the United States. The fear of contagion led to the construction of the State Sanatorium, in 1908, in rural Hoke County, in the sand hills section of the state and miles from the nearest town. Sanatoriums provided state-of-the-art care for tubercular patients while removing them from the general public to prevent transmission of the disease (Futch, 2007). The fear of contagion was a primary reason the state opened Negro Division at the State Sanatorium

15 years later. The *Lenoir News-Topic* announced: "The colored division of the North Carolina Sanatorium was opened in October, 1923.... Tuberculosis is more common among Negroes in North Carolina than among whites" ("Good work," 1924, p. 9). An article in the 1934–36 Biennial Report of the State Sanatorium explained:

> Since Negroes are nurse maids, cooks, food handlers, and personal servants in other capacities in the homes of the white population, their tuberculosis problem also vitally concerns the white people of our State, not only in a humanitarian sense, but also for their own safety. One of the greatest sources of infection among the whites is the Negro servant [Biennial report, 1936, p. 11].

The facility opened with 64 beds, half for women and half for men. The African American patients were treated by the same white physicians who treated the white patients. African Americans with tuberculosis often waited nine month or more for admission to the facility. The 1934–36 Biennial Report of the North Carolina State Sanatorium reported:

> The greatly crowded and unhygienic condition under which most Negroes have to live, make it almost impossible for those who are sick to take sufficient precautions to keep from infecting the other members of the household. Such conditions make the shortage of beds for Negroes all the more tragic. There should be at least one sanatorium bed for each of the eleven hundred Negro deaths. Last year we increased our capacity by twenty-five ... but this gives us only one hundred and fifty beds for Negroes. We are running several months behind with our applications for both men and women Negro patients. As a result, more than 90% are in the advanced stage and many of them in a hopeless condition by the time they are admitted [p. 11].

Treatment lasted six months to two years and consisted of strict regimens of rest, a diet with a lot of milk and meat from the hospital's dairy, and, in some cases, surgery. The extent of racial segregation in state-supported health care facilities is illustrated by an interesting item that appeared in the January 15, 1927, newspaper, *The Robesonian* of Lumberton. The article titled "Indian tubercular patients may get separate quarters" details a plan for the construction of separate beds for the state's Native Americans in the State Sanatorium. It reads in part: "Construction has just begun on a sanatorium annex ... several private rooms for use by the Indians would be available in about a year. At present, the Indians are cared for in the colored hospital division" ("Indian tubercular patients," 1927, p. 1). Effective medications to treat tuberculosis were developed in the 1950s and 1960s, making placement in a sanatorium unnecessary for most people. The State Sanatorium integrated in 1965 to comply with the *Simkins v. Moses H. Cone* court decision and the Civil Rights Act of 1964. The facility remained open until 1983 treating people with intransigent cases of tuberculosis. The State Sanatorium facilities were transferred to the state prison system and is still in use as a prison hospital (Futch, 2007).

Mrs. Carrie Early Broadfoot was the first Head Nurse of the Negro

Appendix I

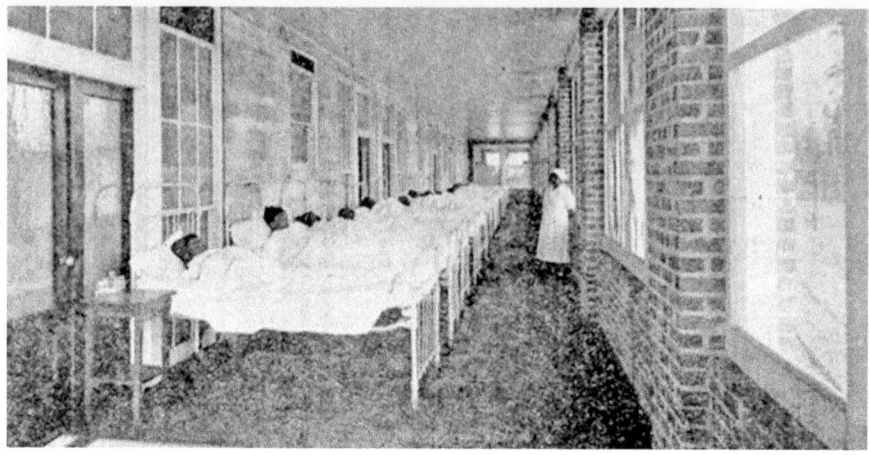

The Men's Ward, Negro Division, State Tuberculosis Santatorium, Santatorium. *North Carolina's Social Welfare Program for Negroes*, special bulletin issued by the North State Board of Charities and Public Welfare, Raleigh, North Carolina, 1923.

Division of the State Sanatorium. Mrs. Broadfoot was born June 13, 1870, in Virginia, and educated at Frederick Douglass Memorial Hospital School of Nursing in Philadelphia. She graduated in 1899 and served as nursing Superintendent of that hospital from 1900 to 1904. In 1905, Broadfoot moved to North Carolina to become the Superintendent of Nurses at St. Agnes Hospital in Raleigh. She joined the American Red Cross and planned to go overseas during World War I to serve in the U.S. Army nurse corps. Instead she was directed to work at home to help control the influenza epidemic sweeping the country. After the influenza crisis passed, Broadfoot became a private duty nurse in Fayetteville until she was invited to become the Superintendent of the new Negro Divisions at the State Sanatorium in Hoke County in 1923. In addition to directing the nursing care at the Sanatorium, in 1925 she organized and then directed the two-year North Carolina Sanatorium Training School for Negro Nurses. The first two graduates were Clareta Redding and Mary Elliott.

Broadfoot directed the Negro Division of the State Sanatorium and its school of nursing until she suffered a stroke in 1943. She had a difficult recovery and her failing health forced her to give up her position. By that time, she was widowed, so she moved to Boston to be cared for by her sister. Broadfoot died January 6, 1945. When Mrs. Broadfoot left the State Sanatorium, the Board of Directors issued this resolution:

> The Board of Directors of the North Carolina Sanatorium learns with deep regret of the sickness of Mrs. Carrie E. Broadfoot and desires to express their earnest wish for her speedy and complete recovery. For twenty years, Mrs.

Broadfoot has been the Superintendent of Nurses of the Negro of the North Carolina Sanatorium and she has labored unceasingly and oftentimes at the expense of her health for the welfare of the institution. We were exceedingly fortunate in securing her services in the organization of the North Carolina Sanatorium Training School for Negro Nurses, the second Tuberculosis Training School in the United States. Her outstanding ability, splendid character and lofty ideals and her prestige as organizer of the Negro State Nurses Association of North Carolina in 1923 and as president for the first eight years and as recording secretary of the National Association of Negro Nurses have done much in establishing the Sanatorium and the Training School in the confidence of the Negroes over the State and in getting them to take advantage of the facilities offered for the treatment and prevention of tuberculosis. Be it resolved that the Board of Directors of the North Carolina Sanatorium express their appreciation for the outstanding services Mrs. Broadfoot has rendered the institution and the cause of tuberculosis in the state [Mrs. Carrie E. Broadfoot, 1944, p. 2].

Negro Division State Orthopedic Hospital, 1926–1966

On July, 1, 1921, North Carolina joined Massachusetts, New York, California, and Michigan to become the fifth State to open a tax-supported hospital for crippled children. Major widespread diseases, primarily tuberculosis and polio, deformed the bones and joints of hundreds of children across the state. Most physicians were in general practice and did not have the knowledge or facilities to treat this specialized group of patients. In the 1921–1923 budget, state lawmakers appropriated 100,000 for the orthopedic hospital. When the hospital opened, it consisted of the administration building, a 50-bed dormitory, cottages for the surgeons, the nurses, and a caretaker as well as a barn on 26 rolling acres in Gaston County. Although the buildings and grounds were paid for by African American as well as white tax dollars, only white children were admitted (North Carolina Orthopedic Hospital, 2016).

There was also a great need for orthopedic care among the state's African American children. Instead of looking to the taxpayers to meet this need, Mrs. Kate Burr Johnson, the state commissioner of public welfare, asked James B. Duke, of the philanthropic Duke family, to donate enough funds to build a wooden 25-bed Negro ward at the orthopedic hospital and staff it for a year. Mrs. Johnson hoped that the state legislature would then take over financial responsibility for the Negro ward ("Mr. Duke Gives," 1925). In 1925, after Mr. Duke made his donation, the state purchased six acres adjoining the Orthopedic Hospital and used Mr. Duke's money to erect and supply the ward. The Benjamin N. Duke Pavilion for Colored Children opened on March 4, 1926. All of the beds were immediately filled with African American children who had been on a waiting list. Recognizing the wooden building was a fire hazard, hospital officials asked Mr. Duke's heirs to give another $25,000 to construct a fireproof 50-bed dormitory for African American children. The old building would then be used as an office and nurse's dormitory for the African American division of the hospital. Mr. Duke's heirs agree to this request (McBryde & Spence, 1991). Mr. Robert Babbington, President of the Orthopedic Hospital, wrote to Mr. Duke's heirs:

> There are twenty boys and six girls in the [1925] cottage today. Every bed has been filled every day since it opened. We have 34 Negro children on the waiting list now. Since the opening of this ward, 171 children have been fully corrected or materially benefitted able to return to their homes able to play and work as normal children.... This $25,000 comes as a Godsend. We will now be able to house our Negro children in a beautiful, fireproof building, increasing our bed facilities to fifty, thus enabling us to do a larger work [as cited in McBryde & Spence, 1991, p. 9].

The new facility opened on November 22, 1930. African American and white patients used the same operating and treatment rooms but were segregated in their housing and schooling. There were separate wings of the white dormitory for male and female patients. However, the Duke Pavilion was not large enough to have two wings and all the children lived with little regard for gender privacy (Healing the children, n.d.).

In 1965, after the 1963 *Simkins v. Moses H. Cone* court decision and the enactment to the Civil Rights Act of 1964, the Gaston County chapter of the National Association for the Advancement of Colored People (NAACP) investigated the orthopedic hospital to check for compliance with the new integration mandates. They issued a news release on March 2, 1966, with their findings:

> The living facilities of this hospital are segregated according to race.... Negro patients are housed in a building which is separate from the main building and joined by an unheated ramp.... Because of the limited facilities in the Negro Building, the separation of the children on the basis of sex, for all age groups, is impossible. This condition does not prevail in the white sections [as cited in McBryde & Spence, 1991, p. 39].

In addition, the NAACP committee found racial segregation in staffing with all 10 teachers being white and nurses of each race only caring for children of their own race. There were no African American physicians on the staff. Officials of the orthopedic hospital were ignoring both the *Simkins V. Moses H Cone* court decision and the Civil Rights Act of 1964 ("NAACP requests," 1966). The Gaston County chapter of the NAACP involved the Office of Equal Health Opportunity, the enforcement division for the Civil Rights Act of 1964 for all medical matters, and within months, the North Carolina Orthopedic Hospital became fully integrated. The hospital continued to serve orthopedically impaired children of North Carolina until 1979 when medical advances made the facility unnecessary (McBryde & Spence, 1991).

Appendix II
Timeline of Significant Events Related to African American Hospitals in North Carolina, 1865–1965

1865—United States General Hospital for Colored Troops opened in Wilmington.
April 1865—Union occupation forces integrated the state psychiatric Dix Hospital in Raleigh.
1866–1869—Eight Freedman's Bureau hospitals provided hospital care for newly freed African Americans.
1880—The tax-supported, segregated North Carolina Asylum for the Colored Insane opened in Goldsboro, for the treatment of African Americans with mental illness. It currently operates as the integrated Cherry Hospital.
1882—Leonard Medical School (LMS), the only African American medical school in North Carolina and the first four-year medical school in the United States, opened in Raleigh. It closed in 1914.
1885—Leonard Hospital, the first general hospital for African Americans in North Carolina, which also served as the clinical training facility for LMS students, opened in Raleigh. It closed in 1914.
1887—The Old North State Medical Society, one of the oldest medical societies for African American physicians in the United States, was established by Lawson A. Scruggs, James T. Williams, Manassa T. Pope, and Aaron McDuffie Moore, graduates of Leonard Medical School.
1887—The Union/Colored Hospital opened in Charlotte, under the auspices of a group of local African American and White women. It closed in 1904.
1891—Good Samaritan Hospital opens in Charlotte. It closed in 1960.
1896—In the *Plessy v. Ferguson* case, the U.S. Supreme Court ruled that states may pass laws imposing racial segregation in public accommodations such as schools, libraries, parks and hospitals. Segregated

facilities were legal if they were separate but of equal in quality to their white counterparts.

1896—St. Agnes Hospital and School of Nursing—the first nursing school for African Americans in North Carolina, opened in Raleigh. It closed in 1961.

1896—Dr. L.A. Scruggs opened the Pickford Sanitarium for treating African Americans with tuberculosis in Southern Pines. It closed in 1912.

1901—Lincoln Hospital opened in Durham. It closed as did Watts Hospital (white) in 1976 when Durham County General Hospital opened.

1902—Slater Hospital opened in Winston, it closed around 1912.

1905—Dr. Hargrave's Hospital opened in Wilson. It evolved into Wilson Hospital and Tubercular Home in 1913 and closed in 1927.

1910—Torrence Hospital opened in Asheville. It closed with Dr. Torrence's death in 1915.

1912—Circle Terrace Sanatorium opened in Asheville. It closed around 1917.

1913—Wilson Hospital and Tubercular Home opened in Wilson. It closed in 1927.

1913—Williamson Sanatorium opened in Winston-Salem. It closed by 1917.

1914—Cordice Sanitarium opened in Greensboro. It closed in 1918, when Dr. Cordice joined other physicians to establish the larger Trinity Hospital.

1918—Trinity Hospital opened in Greensboro. It closed in 1927 when L. Richardson Hospital opened.

1919—The Colored Hospital opened in Oxford. It closed the same year.

1920—Ray's Hospital opened in Winston-Salem. It closed in 1925.

1920—Community Hospital opened in Wilmington. It closed in 1967.

1920—Dr. Erwin's Hospital opened in Gastonia. It closed in 1937.

Early 1920s—Rivera Clinic opened in Mount Olive. It closed in 1965.

1922—Blue Ridge Hospital and School of Nursing opened in Asheville. It closed in 1928.

1923—McCauley Private Hospital opened in Raleigh. It closed in 1961.

1923—The Negro Division of the State Sanitarium opened in Sanitarium. It closed as a separate facility in 1965 when, the state complied with the Civil Rights Act and African American patients were housed, treated and ate with white patients.

1924—The Duke Endowment was established. One of its purposes was to improve health care of low-income people in North and South Carolina, primarily through donating money to underwrite charity care. Several African American hospitals in North Carolina benefited from the Endowment's largess for several decades.

1924—St. Frances Hospital opened in Greenville. It closed in 1934.

1925—The segregated Davis Hospital in Statesville opened a "Negro Branch" in the home of Nurse Daisy Robinson.

1926—Bigelow Hospital opened in Laurinburg on the campus of Laurinburg Institute. It closed in the 1940s.

1926—The Negro Division of the State Orthopedic Hospital (the Duke

Pavilion) opened. It merged with the white division of the facility in 1965–1966.
1927—L. Richardson Hospital opened in Greensboro. It closed in 1985.
1927—Susie Cheatham Hospital opened in Oxford. It closed in 1953 when Shaw Memorial Hospital opened.
1927—Wilson Colored Hospital opened in Wilson. It closed in 1929.
1929—Dr. Furlonge's hospital opened in Smithfield. It closed in 1951.
1937—Gaston County Colored Hospital opened in 1937. It closed in 1966.
1939—Good Shepherd Hospital opened in New Bern. It closed in 1966.
1941—Shuford Clinic opened in Asheville. It closed in 1943.
1943—Asheville Colored Hospital opened in Asheville. It closed in 1951.
1946—Quigless Clinic opened in Tarboro. It closed in 1974.
1946—The U.S. Congress passed the Hospital Survey and Construction Act, better known as the Hill-Burton Act, providing federal funds for hospital construction and improvements. The goal was to achieve a ratio of one general hospital bed for every 4.5 citizens in each state. The Act funded 27 white-only and four African American hospital projects in North Carolina before funding segregated facilities with Hill-Burton funds became illegal in 1963.
1949—The North Carolina Nurse Association merged with the North Carolina Negro Nurse Association, forming one of the first integrated professional organizations in North Carolina.
1950—Leary-Perry Hospital for Mothers and Newborns opened in Fayetteville. It closed the same year.
1953—Shaw Memorial Hospital opened in Oxford. It closed in 1967.
1956—Dr. Hubert Eaton, Dr. Daniel Roane and others sued the segregated James Walker Memorial Hospital in Wilmington over the denial of staff privileges for African American physicians. They lost.
1962—Dr. George Simkins, a Greensboro dentist led a lawsuit against Moses H. Cone Memorial Hospital and Wesley Long Hospital over segregated hiring and admission policies. They won in 1963.
1964—The U.S. Congress passed the Civil Rights Act of 1964 mandating racial equality in facilities receiving public funds.
1965—The U.S. Congress passed additions to the Social Security Act of 1935 known as Medicare, medical insurance for those over 65, and Medicaid, medical insurance for low income Americans. When threatened with the loss of these funds, many hospitals in North Carolina and across the south, enforced race-blind hiring and admission policies.
1965—The North Carolina Medical Society voted to allow African American physicians to become full members. However, the North Carolina Medical Society (white) and the Old North State Medical Society (African American) never merged.

Appendix III
42 Public and Private African American Hospitals in North Carolina, 1880–1967

*=Nursing School (Yes, No)

Name of Hospital	Town/County	NS*	Dates	Sponsored by
1 Cherry (Psychiatric Hospital)	Goldsboro/Wayne	N	August 1, 1880–1965	State Institution
2 Leonard Hospital	Raleigh/Wake	N	1885–1914	White Baptists
3 Union/Colored Hospital	Charlotte/Mecklenburg	N	1887–1894	Local women—interracial
4 Good Samaritan Hospital	Charlotte/Mecklenburg	Y	Sept 23, 1891–1982	White Protestant Episcopal Church
5 St. Agnes Hospital	Raleigh/Wake	Y	Oct. 18, 1896–1961	White Episcopal Church
6 Pickford Sanitarium	Southern Pines/Moore	N	1897–1913	African American physician
7 Lincoln Hospital	Durham/Durham	Y	1901–1976	African American physicians/Washington Duke, philanthropist
8 Slater Hospital	Winston-Salem/Forsyth	N	1902—circa 1912	Slater Institute leaders/R.J. Reynolds, philanthropist
9 Dr. Hargrave's Hospital	Wilson/Wilson	N	1905–1913	African American physician
10 Torrence Hospital	Asheville/Buncombe	N	1910–1915	African American physician
11 Jubilee Hospital	Henderson/Vance County	Y	1911–1966	White Presbyterian Women's Home Missionary Organiztion

Public and Private Hospitals, 1880–1967

Name of Hospital	Town/County	NS*	Dates	Sponsored by
12 Circle Terrace Sanatorium	Asheville/Buncombe	N	1912–1917	African American physician
13 Quality Hill Sanitarium	Monroe/Union	N	1912–1940s	African American physician
14 Mercy Hospital and Tubercular Home	Wilson/Wilson	N	1913–mid-1920s	African American physician and community leaders
15 Williamson Sanatorium	Winston-Salem/Forsyth	N	1914–1917	African American physician
16 Cordice Sanitarium	Greensboro/Guildford	N	1914–1918	African American physician
17 Rivera Clinic	Mount Olive/Wayne	N	1916–1965	African American physician
18 Trinity Hospital	Greensboro/Guilford	N	1918–1927	African American physician
19 Colored Hospital	Oxford/Granville	N	1919–1920	African American nurse
20 Dr. Erwin's Hospital	Gastonia/Gaston	N	1920–1937	African American physician
21 Community Hospital	Wilmington/New Hanover	Y	Sept. 29, 1920–1967	African American physicians
22 Ray's Hospital	Winston-Salem/Forsyth	N	1920–1925	African American physician
23 Blue Ridge Hospital	Asheville/Buncombe	Y	1922–1930	African American Community
24 McCauley Private Hospital	Raleigh/Wake	Y	1923–1950s	African American physician
25 St. Frances Hospital	Greenville/Pitt	N	1924–1933	African American Nurse Frances Hopkins/County government
26 Negro Division of the State Sanitarium	Sanitarium/Hoke	Y	1924–1960s	State Institution
27 Colored Branch of Davis Hospital	Statesville/Iredell	N	Circa 1925–1940	White administrators of Davis Hospital and African American Nurse Daisy Robinson
28 Negro Unit of State Orthopedic Hospital	Dallas/Gaston	N	1925–1966	State Institution made possible by a gift from Mr. Angier Duke
20 Bigelow Hospital	Laurinburg/Scotland	N	1926–1940s	Laurinburg Institute
30 Susie Cheatham Memorial Hospital	Oxford/Granville	N	1927–1950	African American Physicians

Appendix III

Name of Hospital	Town/County	NS*	Dates	Sponsored by
31 L. Richardson Memorial Hospital	Greensboro/ Guilford	Y	May 18, 1927–1974	African American physicians/ Lunsford Richardson family, philanthropists
32 Wilson Colored Hospital	Wilson/Wilson	N	1927–1929	African American private citizen
33 Dr. Furlonge's Hospital	Smithfield/ Johnston	N	1929–1951	African American physician
34 Mercy Hospital	Wilson/Wilson	N	1930–1965	White physicians
35 Good Shepherd Hospital	New Bern/Craven	N	1937–1966	African American physicians/ Episcopal Church/Duke Endowment/ Rosenwald Fund
36 Gaston County Colored Hospital	Gastonia/Gaston	N	1937–1966	Gaston County/ Duke Endowment
37 Kate B. Reynolds Memorial Hospital	Winston-Salem/ Forsyth	Y	1938–1974	African American physicians/ W.N. Reynolds, philanthropist
38 Shuford Clinic	Asheville/ Buncombe	N	1941–1943	White, female physician Dr. Polly Shuford
39 Asheville Colored Hospital/Victoria Wing of Mission Hospital	Asheville/ Buncombe	N	1943– mid–1960s	Citizens of Asheville led by the Asheville Rotary Club
40 Quigless Clinic	Tarboro/ Edgecombe	N	1946–1965	African American physician
41 Leary-Peary Hospital	Fayetteville/ Cumberland	N	1950	African American physician
42 Shaw Memorial Hospital	Oxford/Granville	N	1953–1967	African American Physician

References

About the colored hospital. (1891, March 9). *The Charlotte News*, p. 1.
Action (n.d.). [Clipping from *The Rotary Cog*, a Rotary Club magazine]. Rotary Club Headquarters, Asheville, NC.
Adams, E. J. (1961). Jubilee Hospital. *Women's Missionary Magazine. 75*(3). p. 798.
Aid for Negro hospital. (1915, January 11). *Greensboro Daily News*, p. 5.
Alexander, K. (1947, October 27). Gaston Negro Hospital fares O.K. but could do with a little more help. *The Gastonia Gazette*, p. 10.
American Medical Association. (1909). *American medical dictionary: A register of legally qualified physicians of the United States and Canada*. Chicago: American Medical Association Press.
Ancestry.com (2016). *U.S., World War II Cadet Nursing Corps Card Files, 1942–1948* [database online]. Provo, UT: Ancestry.com Operations, Inc., 2011.
Anderson, J. B., & Historic Preservation Society of Durham. (1990). *Durham County: A history of Durham County, North Carolina*. Durham: Duke University Press.
Anti-tuberculosis clinics for Gaston. (1920, June 10). *The Gastonia Daily Gazette*, p. 1.
An appeal for the colored hospital. (1891, March 10). *The Charlotte News*, p. 4.
Arnett, E. S. (1955). *Greensboro, North Carolina: The county seat of Guilford*. Chapel Hill: University of North Carolina Press.
Arnett, E. S. (1975). *The Saura and Keyauwee in the land that became Guilford, Randolph, and Rockingham*. Greensboro, NC: Media.
Association recognizes McCauley Hospital here. (1942, April 26). *Raleigh News and Observer*, p. 10.
Ayanian, J. Z. (1982). *Black Health in Segregated Durham, 1900–1940*. Durham: Duke University Press.
Avant, F. W. (1939). The beginning and growth of the colored Community Hospital of Wilmington, North Carolina. *The Health Bulletin, 53*(3), 12–15.
Baily, M. (1983, July 16). Mercy Hospital: Health care in east Wilson. *Wilson Daily Times*, p. 1-C.
Barbee, C. B. (1927, September 20). The Susie Cheatham Memorial Hospital [Clipping from *The Public Ledger*, an Oxford, NC newspaper]. Granville County Public Library, Oxford, NC.
Baby show, track meet, May pole, for benefit of Greensboro hospital. (1927, June 11). *The New York Age*, p. 9.

Beardsley, E. H. (1986). Good-bye to Jim Crow: The desegregation of southern hospitals. *Bulletin of the History of Medicine, 60*(3), 367–86.

Beardsley, E. H. (1987). *History of neglect: Health care for Blacks and mill workers in the twentieth-century south.* Knoxville: University of Tennessee Press.

Beck, A. H. (2004). The Flexner report and the standardization of American medical education. *Journal of the American Medical Association, 291*(17), 2139–40.

Beckford, G. H. (2011). *Biographical dictionary of American physicians of African ancestry: 1800–1920.* Cherry Hill, NJ: Africana Homestead Legacy Publishers.

Bielakowski, A. M. (2013). *Ethnic and racial minorities in the U.S. military: An encyclopedia.* Santa Barbara, CA: ABC-CLIO, LLC.

Bishop Darst to preside at hospital dedication. (1938, June 26). *The New Bern Sun Journal,* p. 1.

A bit of history: When we had a hospital. (2014, April 16). *Wake Forest Gazette.* Retrieved from: http://wakeforestgazette.com/bit-history-hospital/.

Black Diamond Quartette. (1888, August 2). *The Charlotte Observer,* p. 4.

Black history month. (2009). Retrieved from: http://history.amedd.army.mil/ancwebsite/articles/blackhistory.html.

Blackburn, C. (2006) Making history. *Our State Magazine.* Retrieved from: http://www.shawuniversity.edu/assets/Making_History.pdf.

Blackburn, G. T. (1984). *The heritage of Vance County, North Carolina.* Winston-Salem, NC: Hunter Pub. Co.

Bond, R. (2008). *A town called Dehra.* New Delhi: Penguin Books.

Bricker, M. L. (2008). *Winston-Salem: A twin city history.* Charleston, SC: History Press.

Brown, L. (2008). *Upbuilding Black Durham: Gender, class, and Black community development in the Jim Crow South.* Chapel Hill: University of North Carolina Press.

Building fund drive for Susie Cheatham launched. (1945, October 30). [Clipping from *The Public Ledger,* an Oxford, NC, newspaper]. Granville County Public Library, Oxford, NC.

Byrd, W. M. and Clayton, L. A. (2000). *An American health dilemma: A medical history of African Americans and the problem of race beginnings to 1900, volume 1.* New York: Routledge.

Byrd, W. M. and Clayton, L. A. (2001). *An American health dilemma: A medical history of African Americans and the problem of race beginnings to 1900, volume 2.* New York: Routledge.

Caldwell, A. B. (1921). *History of the American Negro and his institutions.* Atlanta: A. B. Caldwell Publishing Company.

Campbell, E. (1995). "Henderson Institute." Retrieved from: http://www.hpo.ncdcr.gov/nr/VN0019.pdf.

Campbell, K. (2016). History of Good Samaritan Hospital. Retrieved from: http://cityunwrapped.com/history-of-good-samaratin-hospital/.

Cannon, D. (1983, October 18). Seasickness, winter storm led Dr. C.W. Furlonge to Johnston. *The Smithfield Herald,* p. B1.

A card. (1893, December 23). *The Charlotte Observer,* p. 4.

A card of thanks. (1886, December 22). *The Charlotte Observer,* p. 1.

Carlson, A. J., & Brown, M. A. (1988). *The history and architecture of Granville County, North Carolina.* Oxford, NC: Granville Historical Society.

Carr, D. (2009). "Health care in early Wilson: Retrieved from: https://archive.org/stream/trojan19591959char/trojan19591959char_djvu.txt.
Carter, K. M. (1957). *Sampson County MDs*. Clinton, NC: The Commercial Printing Company.
Carter, W. A. (1973). *Shaw's universe: A monument to educational innovation*. Raleigh: Shaw University.
Cartwright, S. (1851). Diseases and peculiarities of the Negro race. *De Bow's Review of Southern and Western States*. Retrieved from http://www.pbs.org/wgbh/aia/part4/4h3106t.html.
Chamber secretary commends hospital. (1922, September 18). *The Wilmington Morning Star*, p. 8.
Chafe, W. H., Gavins, R., & Korstad, R. (2001). *Remembering Jim Crow: African Americans tell about life in the segregated South*. New York: New Press.
Charlotte, N.C. hospital suspends 22 students. (1959, October 29). *Jet Magazine*, p. 52.
Charlotte Chronicle. (1891, May 5). *Wilmington Morning Star*, p. 3.
Cherry Hospital. (1997). Retrieved from: http://www.ncmarkers.com/Markers.aspx?MarkerId=F-61.
Cherry Hospital. (2016). Retrieved from: http://www.asylumprojects.org/index.php?title=Cherry_Hospital.
Christopher, M. (1971). *America's Black congressmen*. New York: Thomas Y. Crowell Company.
The churches work among the Negroes [Brochure]. (1902). Found in the Good Samaritan Collection at the North Carolina State Library, Raleigh, North Carolina.
Cimbala, P. A., & Miller, R. M. (1999). *The Freedmen's Bureau and Reconstruction*. New York: Fordham University Press.
City of Winston-Salem. (2016). City of Winston-Salem history. Retrieved from: http://www.cityofws.org/home-center/discover-winston-salem/city-of-winston-salem-history.
Clement, M. H. (2001). *100 years of caring: The history of Highsmith Hospital School of Nursing*. Fayetteville, NC: Old Mountain Press.
Close doors of Negro Hospital. (1930, August 9). *Asheville Citizen Times*, p. 68.
The closing session of Leonard Medical School. (1887, April 13). *The Biblical Recorder*, p. 2.
Cobb, W. M. (1947). *Medical care and the plight of the Negro*. New York: NAACP.
Cobb, W. M. (1961). Saint Agnes Hospital, Raleigh, North Carolina, 1896–1961. *Journal of the National Medical Association*, 53(5). 439–446.
Cobb, W. M. (1964). The hospital integration story in Charlotte, North Carolina. *Journal of the National Medical Association*, 56 (3), 226–229.
Coffin, L. (1968). *Reminiscences of Levi Coffin*. New York: Arno Press.
Colored committee raises fund. (1943, January 31). *Asheville Citizen Times*, p. A 1–2.
Colored doctors plan to establish hospital. (1916, October 20). *Twin City Daily Sentinel*, p. 5.
Colored folks to celebrate the forth (1919, July 1). *Oxford Public Ledger*, p. 8.
The Colored Hospital. (1888, July 29). *The Charlotte Chronicle*, p. 2.
The Colored Hospital. (1889, February 5). *The Charlotte Observer*, p. 4.
A colored hospital. (1912, July 30). *The Charlotte Observer*, p. 10.
Colored hospital. (1912, October 1). *The High Point Enterprise*, p.1.

References

The Colored Hospital. (1916, December 7). *Greensboro Daily News*, p. 12.
Colored hospital formally opened. (1922, September 29). *Asheville Citizen Times*, p. A-4.
Colored hospital is soon to be realized. (1919, May 19). *The Gastonia Gazette*, p. 8.
Colored hospital movement is growing. (1919, November 22). *The Gastonia Gazette*, p. 8.
Colored hospital nearing completion. (1919, November 29). *The Gastonia Gazette*, p. 8.
Colored hospital nucleus started at 114 N. Wash. Street. (1923, October 22). [Clipping from *The Daily Reflector*, a Greenville, NC, newspaper]. East Carolina University Library, Greenville, NC.
Colored hospital planned for Statesville. (1912, October 1). *The Charlotte News*, p. 7.
Colored hospital to open today for inspection. (1943, October 21). *The Asheville Citizen*, p. B-3.
Colored maternity hospital makes appeal for money. (1950, August 11). *The Fayetteville Observer*, p. 2.
Colored nursing school will open here on January fourth. (1941, December 29). *The Fayetteville Observer*, p. 2.
Colored physician died yesterday. (1915, May 23). *The Asheville Citizen Times*, p. A-6.
Colored tuberculosis hospital open. (1914). *Journal of Outdoor Life*, XI, p. 349.
Colgrove, J. (2002). The McKeown Thesis: A historical controversy and its enduring influence. *American Journal of Public Health*, 92(5), 725–729.
Commissioners give $1,000 for hospital. (1920, January 6). *The Gastonia Gazette*, p. 1.
The Community Hospital. (1923). *Journal of the National Medical Association*. 15(2), 114.
Community Hospital a monument to vision and spirit of sacrifice. (1921, February 28). *The Wilmington Star*, p. 8.
Community hospital to cease operation due to lack of use. (1966, September 28). [Clipping from *The Gastonia Gazette*, a Gastonia, NC newspaper]. Gaston County Public Library, Gastonia, NC.
Conducting campaign for Negro hospital. (1915, September 7). *The Greensboro Daily News*, p. 9.
Conference for the study of the Negro problems. (1896). *Mortality among Negroes in cities: Proceedings of the Conference for Investigation of City Problems, held at Atlanta University, May 26–27, 1896*. Atlanta: Atlanta University Press.
Cordice, Dr. John Walter Vincent. (2012). Retrieved from: http://www.opendurham.org/people/cordice-dr-john-walter-vincent.
Corner stone of Negro hospital is laid on Sunday. (1938, June 28). *The New Bern Sun Journal*, p. 1–2.
County bills ordered paid. (1932, April 8). *The Statesville Landmark*, p. 6.
County ups subsidy for Negro Hospital. (1959, November 10). *The Gastonia Gazette*, p. 8.
Cue, C. B., & Davis, L. G. (2000). *Winston-Salem State University*. Charleston, SC: Arcadia.
Davis, L. G. (1980). *The Black heritage of western North Carolina*. Asheville, NC: Authors.

de Roulhac, H. J. G. (1909). The Freedmen's Bureau in North Carolina. *Southern Atlantic Quarterly, 8,* 53–67.
Death of colored woman. (1918, March 4). *Twin City Daily Sentinel,* p. 12.
Decide to establish hospital for Negroes. (1915, May 11). *The Greensboro Daily News,* p. 3.
Delany, L. T. (1930). St. Agnes Hospital. *Journal of the National Medical Association, 22*(3), 135–136.
Demographics. (2016). In Pitt County. Retrieved from: http://places.mooseroots.com/l/314215/Craven-County-NC.
Demographics. (2016). In Durham County. Retrieved from http://places.mooseroots.com/l/314222/Durham-County-NC.
Demographics. (2016). In Granville County. Retrieved from: http://places.mooseroots.com/l/314229/Granville-County-NC.
Demographics. (2016). In Johnston County. Retrieved from: http://places.mooseroots.com/l/314241/Johnston-County-NC.
Demographics. (2016). In Pitt County. Retrieved from: http://places.mooseroots.com/l/314264/Pitt-County-NC.
Demographics. (2015). In Union County. Retrieved from: http://places.mooseroots.com/l/314280/Union-County-NC.
Discrimination in North Carolina hospitals. (1963). *Journal of the National Medical Association, 55*(1), 57–58.
Dr. A. H. Ray. (1954, October 15). *Twin City Sentinel,* p.1
Dr. C. W. Furlonge dies of heart failure at 85. (1972, June 27). *The Smithfield Herald,* p. B-1.
Dr. John Sherman Massey. (2016). Retrieved from: http://www.findagrave.com/cgi-bin/fg.cgi?page=gr&GRid=84998710.
Dr. L. McCauley, prominent area resident, dies. (1952, March 24). *The Carolina Times,* p. 1.
Dr. Rivera's Clinic. (1930, September 20). *New York Age,* p. 10.
Dr. Thomas Monte Rivera. (1953, May 23). *The Goldsboro News Argus,* p. 7.
Doctor writes autobiography. (1994, May 11). *The Detroit Free Press,* p. 7.
Doctors give funds for Negro hospital. (1945). *Southern Medicine and Surgery, 107,* p. 160.
Doles, D. (1987, September 18). Tarboro didn't need a trombone player. *The Daily Southerner,* p. 1B.
Dorothea Dix Hospital. (2014). The Asylum Project. Retrieved from http://www.asylumprojects.org/index.php?title=Dorothea_Dix_Hospital.
Dudley, G. (1987, September 21). Two days for Dr. M.D. Quigless. *The Daily Southerner,* n.p.
Durden, R. F. (1998). *Lasting legacy to the Carolinas: The Duke Endowment, 1924–1994.* Durham: Duke University Press.
The earliest Negro physicians and colored hospital in Gaston County [Pamphlet]. (n.d.). Found in the Gaston County Public Library.
Eaton, H. A. (1965). Community Hospital, Wilmington, North Carolina. *Journal of the National Medical Association, 57*(1), 74–79.
Eaton, H. A. (1984). *Every man should try.* Wilmington, NC: Bonaparte Press.
Elkins, W. O. (1969). A History of L. Richardson Memorial Hospital. *North Carolina Medical Journal, 30*(4), 146–51.
Embree, E. R., & Waxman, J. (1949). *Investment in people: The story of the Julius Rosenwald Fund.* New York: Harper.

Emerson, A. M. (1913). Leonard Hospital. *Journal of the National Medical Association*, 5(2), 86–89.
English, W. T. (1903). The Negro problem from the physician's point of view. *Atlanta Journal-Record of Medicine*, 5, 461.
Erect race hospital. (1927, January 15). *The Pittsburgh Courier*, p. 1.
Ewbank, D.C. (1987). History of Black mortality and health before 1940. *The Milbank Quarterly*, 65, 100–128.
Exchange Club gives $25 to new hospital. (1950, August 30). *The Fayetteville Observer*, n.p.
Fett, S. M. (2002). *Working cures: Healing, health, and power on southern slave plantations.* Chapel Hill: University of North Carolina Press.
First Graduates. (1925). Record number: bhcP77.10.2.8.1. Heritage of Black Highlanders Collections, Special Collections of the D. H. Ramsey Library, UNC Asheville.
Fisher, J. E. (1986). *The John F. Slater Fund: A nineteenth century affirmative action for Negro education.* Lanham, MD: University Press of America.
Fisher, W. D. & Douglas, J. H. (2016) *African American doctors of World War I: the lives of 104 volunteers.* Jefferson, NC: McFarland.
Flexner, A. (1910) *Medical education in the United States and Canada: A report to the Carnegie foundation for the advancement of teaching.* Carnegie Foundation for the Advancement of Teaching. New York: Carnegie Foundation.
Fleishman, J. (1994, May 30). The long, good fight of Dr. Quigless. *The Philadelphia Inquirer.* Retrieved from: http://articles.philly.com/1994-05-30/news/25829967_1_seat-belt-black-hospital-black-school.
Formal Opening of Colored Hospital. (1922, September 24). *Asheville Citizen Times*, p. 32.
Fort Bragg. (2013). Retrieved from: http://www.bragg.army.mil/Pages/History.aspx.
Funds available for colored hospital here reports. (1919, April 4). *The Public Ledger*, p. 1.
Funeral of Dr. Torrence was held yesterday. (1915, May 26). *The Asheville Gazette-News*, p. 7.
Funeral Thursday for Dairy Robinson. (1947, January 9). *The Statesville Landmark*, p. 16.
Futch, M. (2007, July 7). The TB hospital. *The Fayetteville Observer.* Retrieved from: http://www.fayobserver.com/news/local/the-tb-hospital/article_7da3b228-231a-56a6-9c73-e60e6b505690.html.
Gamble, V. N. (1989). *Germs have no color lines: Blacks and American medicine, 1900–1940.* New York: Garland.
Gamble, V. N. (1995). *Making a place for ourselves: The Black hospital movement, 1920–1945.* New York: Oxford University Press.
Gaston, M. H. (1946, November 13). Negro hospital closes ten years of service this week. [Clipping from *The Gastonia Gazette,* a Gastonia, NC newspaper]. Gaston County Public Library, Gastonia, NC.
Gaston County Museum (n.d.). Medical Case. Retrieved from http://www.gastoncountymuseum.org/objectotw1.31.11.asp.
Gastonia Negro Hospital gets new superintendent Thursday. (1954, June 30). *The Gaston Citizen*, p. 4.
Genealogical Society of Iredell County, NC. (1980). *The heritage of Iredell County, 1980.* Statesville, NC: Genealogical Society of Iredell County.
Giri, V. (2014) "To collect their shattered energies": Hammond Hospital and mil-

itary mental healthcare during the Civil War. *Armstrong Undergraduate Journal of History, 4*(2), 1.
Godwin, J. L. (2000). *Black Wilmington and the North Carolina way: Portrait of a community in the era of civil rights protest.* Lanham, MD: University Press of America.
Golden rule class sews for infants. (1963, November 6). *The Standard-Speaker,* p. 14.
The Good Samaritan. (1888, December 19). *The Charlotte Observer,* p. 4.
Good Samaritan Hospital. (1892). *Annual report of the Good Samaritan Hospital.* Charlotte, NC: Good Samaritan Hospital.
Good Samaritan Hospital. (1903). *Twelfth annual report of the Good Samaritan Hospital.* Charlotte, NC: Good Samaritan Hospital.
Good Samaritan Hospital. (1948). *Be a good Samaritan* [Brochure]. Found in the North Carolina State library, Raleigh, NC.
Good Shepherd Hospital. (1938, June 12). *The New Bern Sun Journal,* p. 1.
A good work in charity that needs help. (1889, March 26). *The Charlotte News,* p. 3.
Good work of the State Colored Sanatorium (1924, December 18). *The Lenoir News-Topic,* p. 9.
Great Interest. (1904, February 27). *Winston-Salem Journal,* p. 1.
Greensboro Historical Museum. (2016). *Lunsford Richardson.* Retrieved from: http://archives.greensborohistory.org/manuscripts/smith-family.
Greenwood, J. (1994). *Bittersweet legacy: The black and white "better classes" in Charlotte 1850–1910.* Chapel Hill: University of North Carolina Press.
Grimes, M. S. (1972). The history of Kate Bitting Reynolds Memorial Hospital. *Journal of the National Medical Association.* 64(4), 376–381.
Grob, G. N. (1994). *The mad among us: A history of the care of America's mentally ill.* New York: Free Press.
Grundy, E. (2005). Commentary: The McKeown debate: Time for burial. *International Journal of Epidemiology, 34*(3), 529–533.
Hairston, L. (1903). "Slater Hospital" in the 1903 North Carolina Board of Public Charities Biennial Report for 1901–1902. Raleigh, NC: Edwards and Broughton State Printers.
Haller, J. S. (1971). *Outcasts from evolution: Scientific attitudes of racial inferiority, 1859–1900.* Urbana: University of Illinois Press.
Halliburton, C. D. (1937). *A history of St. Augustine's College, 1867–1937.* Raleigh, NC: St. Augustine College.
Halperin, E. C. (1988). Desegregation of Hospitals and Medical Societies in North Carolina. *New England Journal of Medicine, 318*(1), 58–63.
Harris, V. (1996, February 27). Town's first black doctor tells his story. *The Daily Southerner,* p. 1 & 8.
Hartshorn, W.N., & Penniman, G.W. (1910). *An era of progress and promise, 1863–1910: The religious, moral and educational development of the American Negro since his emancipation.* Boston: Priscilla Publishing Company.
Hawkins, O. W. (2008). *Pickford Sanitarium and R.C. Lawson Institute: Two former institutions of Southern Pines, North Carolina.* Southern Pines, NC: Author.
Healing the children. (n.d.). Retrieved from: http://www.gastoncountymuseum.org/PDF/healing.pdf.
Hemmingway, T. (1980). Prelude to change: Black Carolinians in the war years, 1914–1920. *Journal of Negro History, 65,* 212–227.

Henderson Hospital. (1921). *Women's Missionary Magazine 35*(3), 177.
Henderson, N.C. (1916). *Women's Missionary Magazine 29*(8), 797–799.
Heritage of Johnston County Book Committee. (1985). *The heritage of Johnston County, North Carolina, 1985.* Winston-Salem, NC: Published by the Heritage of Johnston County Book Committee in cooperation with the History Division, Hunter Pub. Co.
Hine, D. C. (1989). *Black women in white: Racial conflict and cooperation in the nursing profession, 1890–1950.* Bloomington: Indiana University Press.
Historic marker program. (2016). Retrieved from: http://www.cityofws.org/Portals/0/pdf/Planning/HRC/historic-marker-program/Marker-Sheets/26_Kate_Bitting_Reynolds_Memorial_Hospital.pdf.
History. (2013) In *Tuscarora Nation of North Carolina.* Retrieved from: http://www.tuscaroranationnc.com/history.
Hoover, E., & Lewis, C. (2009). Good Samaritan Hospital and the North Carolina Medical College circa early 1900: The first major affiliation between a Black hospital and a white medical college. *Journal of the National Medical Association, 101*(4), 377–381.
The hospital for colored people. (1887, March 13). *The Charlotte Chronicle*, p. 4.
Hospital for colored people meeting with success. (1915, June 22). *The Greensboro Daily News*, p. 10.
Hospital for Negroes grows rapidly here. (1951, September 28). *The Gastonia Gazette*, p. 28.
Hospital given Board support. (1959, October 14). *The Statesville Record and Landmark*, p. 8.
Hospital refuses dying A&T student. (1950, December 9). *Durham Carolina Times*, p. 1.
Hotz, A. (2007, November 9). The lost tribe. *The Wilmington Star.* Retrieved from: http://www.starnewsonline.com/article/20071109/ARTICLE/71108010?p=6&tc=pg.
House of Healing in North Carolina. (1963). *Report to the Board of National Mission, United Presbyterian Church.* Found in the Presbyterian Archives, Philadelphia, PA.
Huffman, W. H., & Hanchett, T. W. (1985) in Morrill, D's *Report to the Charlotte-Mecklenburg Historical Properties Commission.* Retrieved from: http://www.cmhpf.org/S&Rs%20Alphabetical%20Order/surveys&rgoodsam.htm.
Hughes, R. A. H. (1988). *Contributions of Vance County people of color.* Raleigh, NC: Sparks Press.
Hulth, P. (1963, October 18). At 76 Dr. Furlonge is oldest practicing physician in county. *The Smithfield Herald*, p. 1.
Humphreys, M. (2013). *Marrow of tragedy: The health crisis of the American Civil War.* Baltimore: Johns Hopkins University Press.
Hurd, H. M. (1916). *The institutional care of the insane in the United States and Canada, Volume 3.* Baltimore: Johns Hopkins University Press.
Hutchinson, V. (2002). *New Bern.* Charleston, SC: Arcadia Press.
In training: Nursing education in New Hanover County 1901–1066. (2004). Retrieved from: http://library.uncw.edu/web/collections/intraining/CommunityHospital.html.
Indian tubercular patients may get separate quarters. (1937, January, 15). *The Robesonian*, p. 2.
Interesting exercises. (1900, February 10). *The Morning Post*, p. 5.

Jackson, V. (2001). Separate and unequal: The legacy of racially segregated psychiatric hospitals—a cultural competence training tool. Retrieved from: https://www.patdeegan.com/sites/default/files/files/separate_and_unequal.pdf.
Jacobs, C. (2013, July 21). The peaceful revolution. *The Fayetteville Observer*, p. A 1, 4,& 5.
Jeffers, M. M. (1946, December 30). Dr. H. J. Erwin, Negro physician dies, ill 18 months. *Gastonia Gazette*, p. 1.
Jimison, R. (1962, May 23). Gaston Negro Hospital goes modern. *The Gastonia Gazette*, p. A-9.
Johnson, K. T. & Murray, E. R. (2008). *Wake: Capital county of North Carolina. Volume II*. Durham, NC: Maple-Vail Book Manufacturing Group.
Johnson, R. (1939). Report to the Convention on the Good Samaritan Hospital. Minutes of the Episcopal Diocese of East Carolina.
Johnson, R. (1940). Report to the Convention on the Good Samaritan Hospital. Minutes of the Episcopal Diocese of East Carolina.
Johnson, R. (1941). Report to the Convention on the Good Samaritan Hospital. Minutes of the Episcopal Diocese of East Carolina.
Johnson, R. (1950). Report to the Convention on the Good Samaritan Hospital. Minutes of the Episcopal Diocese of East Carolina.
Jones, H. G., Jones, K. R., & Jones, C. D. (2004). *Scoundrels, rogues, and heroes of the Old North State*. Charleston, SC: History Press.
Keever, H. (1974, April 8). Despite meager start, hospital growth evident. *Statesville Record and Landmark*, p. D 1–2.
Krammerer, R. (1986, February 5). A history of the first Pitt County Hospital. *The Greenville Times*, p. 12–13.
L. Richardson Memorial Hospital. (1935) *Annual report of the L. Richardson Memorial Hospital and L. Richardson Memorial Hospital School of Nursing*. Found in the North Carolina Collection, Wilson Library, UNC-Chapel Hill.
LaNey, I. C. (2000). Women and interracial cooperation in establishing the Good Samaritan Hospital. *AFFILIA, 15*(1), 65–81.
Larkin, J. R. (1957). *The Negro population of North Carolina, 1945–1955*. Retrieved from: http://digital.ncdcr.gov/cdm/ref/collection/p249901coll22/id/283128.
Lassiter, T. J., Lassiter, W., & Lassiter, T. J. (2004). *Johnston County: Its history since 1746*. Smithfield, NC: Hometown Heritage Publishing Company.
The Laurinburg Normal and Industrial Institute. (April, 1949). *The Eastern Searchlight 19*(10), 2.
Laurinburg, NC. (1926, November 20). *New York Age*, p. 7.
Laurinburg, NC. (1927, February 19). *New York Age*, p. 9.
Laurinburg, NC. (1927, December 24). *New York Age*, p. 2.
Laurinburg, NC. (1928, August 11). *New York Age*, p. 9.
Laurinburg, NC. (1929, December 24). *New York Age*, p. 2.
Laurinburg, NC. (1931, July 30). *New York Age*, p. 7.
Laurinburg, North Carolina. (1935, September 14). *New York Age*, p. 11.
Laying the cornerstone. (1888. December 21). *The Charlotte Democrat*, p. 3.
Lefler, L. J. (2009). *Under the Rattlesnake: Cherokee Health and Resiliency*. Tuscaloosa: University of Alabama Press.
Leonard Medical School. (1886, October 1). *The African Examiner*, p. 2.
Leonard Medical School catalog, 1907–1908. (1908). Raleigh, NC: Edwards & Broughton Printing Company. Retrieved from https://archive.org/stream/shawuniversityli19081910/shawuniversityli19081910_djvu.txt.

Lewis, J. D. (2013). A history of Wilson County. Retrieved from: http://www.carolana.com/NC/Counties/wilson_county_nc.html.

Lewis, N. (1998). Mercy Hospital: Emergence of the first Black hospital in eastern North Carolina, 1912–1964. (Unpublished Master's Thesis). North Carolina Central University, Durham, NC.

Lewis, R. H. (1897). Health. *The Southern Sanitarium, 1*(1), 18–19. Retrieved from http://docsouth.unc.edu/nc/scruggs/scruggs.html.

Life expectancy in the U.S. (1998). Retrieved from: http://demog.berkeley.edu/~andrew/1918/figure2.html.

Lillard, S. (n.d.). *Good Samaritan Hospital (for Colored people), Charlotte, Mecklenburg County, N.C. 1888/1891–1960/1961*. [Finding aid for the Good Samaritan Collection at the University of North Carolina at Charlotte, NC]. Atkins Library, Charlotte, NC.

Lincoln Hospital linen day drive nets $481.90; Queen crowned. (1961, August 5). *The Carolina Times*, p. 3.

Linder, F. E., & Grove, R. D. (1947). *Vital statistics rates in the United States 1900–1940*, Washington, D.C.: U.S. Government Printing Office.

The local Kiwanis club fosters color hospital for city. (1924, August 9). [Clipping from *The Daily Reflector*, a Greenville, NC newspaper]. East Carolina University Library, Greenville, NC.

Local Negro hospital needs financial aid. (1920, May 3). *Greensboro Daily News*, p. 8.

Lofton, H. (2004, May 26). Interviewed by L. Mims. Randall Library Oral History Collection. University of North Carolina at Wilmington. Retrieved from: http://digitalcollections.uncw.edu/cdm/singleitem/collection/oralhistory/id/450/rec/1.

London, L. F., Lemmon, S. M. C., & Episcopal Church. (1987). *The Episcopal Church in North Carolina, 1701–1959*. Raleigh, NC: Episcopal Diocese of North Carolina.

Long, D. (Ed). (1972). *Medicine in North Carolina; Essays in the history of medical science and medical service, 1524–1960*. Raleigh, NC: North Carolina Medical Society.

Long, G. (2012). *Doctoring freedom: The politics of African American medical care in slavery and emancipation*. Chapel Hill: University of North Carolina Press.

Luck, T. (2012, August 1). Legacy of "Katie B." saluted. *The Winston-Salem Chronicle*. Retrieved from: http://www.wschronicle.com/2012/08/legacy-of-katie-b-saluted/.

Lunsford, B. (2013). *Charlotte: Then and now*. London: Pavilion Book Publishers.

Mangus, A. K. (2015). Dr. Equality. *The Wrightsville Beach Magazine*. Retrieved from: http://wrightsvillebeachmagazine.com/flash/2015-2/#/68/.

Marlowe, N. (2004). *The legacy of Mission Hospital*. Asheville, NC: Mission Hospital.

Massey, John S., M.D. (2012) Pamphlet located in the Dickerson Genealogy and Local History Room of the Union County Public Library in Monroe, North Carolina.

Massey, J. S. (1912, March 26). Dr. Massey asks for aid. *The Monroe Journal*, p. 1.

Maternity home granted charter. (1949, October 6). *The Fayetteville Observer*. [Clipping from *The Fayetteville Observer* a Fayetteville, NC newspaper]. Cumberland County Public Library, Fayetteville, NC.

Mattson, R. (1988). The evolution of Raleigh's African American neighborhoods in the 19th and 20th centuries. Retrieved from: http://rhdc.org/sites/default/files/EvolRaleighAfricanAmericanNeigh.pdf.

Maund, A. (1952). *The Untouchables.* New Orleans, LA: Southern Conference Educational Fund.

Mayo, S. C. (1945). *Negro hospital and medical care facilities in North Carolina.* Raleigh: North Carolina Agricultural Experiment Station, State College Station.

McBryde, A. M., & Spence, R. M. B. (1991). *A history of the North Carolina Orthopedic Hospital: A dream come true.* Gastonia, NC: Author.

McCauley, B. (1990, November 6). Masonic group to buy L. Richardson Hospital. *The Greensboro News and Record.* Retrieved from: http://www.greensboro.com/masonic-group-to-buy-l-richardson-hospital/article_db3c9e27-ecd1-5f59-bfb8-ec30f2bbe0bb.html.

The McCauley Private Hospital. (1927, January 15). *New York Age,* p. 7.

McGhee, B. L. (2014). *Our story: The African American presence in Granville County, North Carolina.* Brown Summit, NC: McGhee Publishing Company, Inc.

McKeown, T. (1979). The role of medicine: dream, mirage or nemesis. Oxford, England: Blackwell.

McKinney, C. W. (2010). *Greater freedom: The evolution of the civil rights struggle in Wilson, North Carolina.* Lanham, MD: University Press of America.

McQueen, L. (2014, June 14). Dr. C. Mason Quick. *The Pilot.* Retrieved from: http://www.thepilot.com/opendaily/dr-c-mason-quick/image_3b951f26-f32f-11e3-bf04-0017a43b2370.html.

Medical Society of New Hanover, Brunswick, and Pender Counties., & Poole, J. (1977). *The lonely road: A history of the physicks and physicians of the lower Cape Fear, 1735–1976.* Place of publication not identified: The Society.

Mega, J. L., Mega, L. T., & King, C. Y. (2000). Early women physicians of eastern North Carolina. Lula Disosway, MD, Malene Grant Irons, MD, and Isa Grant, MD. *North Carolina Medical Journal, 61*(3), 146–149.

Merrell, J. H. (1989). *The Indians' new world: Catawbas and their neighbors from European contact through the era of removal.* Chapel Hill: University of North Carolina Press.

Meyers, B. (2000). *History.* Retrieved from: http://www.scotlandcounty.org/history.aspx.

Miller, J. F. (1905). *Report of the State Hospital at Goldsboro.* Raleigh, NC: E.M. Uzzell and Company, State Printers.

Ministered to the community over 50 years. (1970, November 20). *The Smithfield Herald,* p. 6.

Missionary society has picnic Monday. (1947, August 12). *The News-Herald,* p. 11.

Mr. Duke gives $15,000 to aid Negro cripples. (1925, July 2). *The Albemarle Press,* p. 1.

Mitchell, M. F. (1987). A half-century of health care: Raleigh's Rex Hospital, 1894–1944. *North Carolina Historical Review, 64*(2).162–198.

Mitchell, S. (2014). *Mrs. Elenora Mitchell Walker.* Retrieved from: http://www.colorofasheville.net/history/mrs-elenora-mitchell-walker/.

Moore County Heritage Book Committee. (2005). *Moore County heritage, North Carolina.* Waynesville, NC: County Heritage, Incorporated.

Morehouse, H. L. (1890). *H.M. Tupper, D.D: A narrative of twenty-five years'* work in the South, 1865–1890. New York: American Baptist Home Mission Society.

Morrill, D. L., & Historic Charlotte, Inc. (2001). *Historic Charlotte: An illustrated history of Charlotte & Mecklenburg County*. San Antonio, TX: Historical Pub. Network.

Moss, R. J. (2005). *Eden in the pines: A history of Pinehurst Village*. Southern Pines, NC: The Pilot.

Murray, E. R. (1983). *Wake, capital county of North Carolina*. Raleigh, NC: Capital County Publishing Company.

Murray, E. R. (1996). "L.A. Scruggs" in *Dictionary of North Carolina biography*, William S. Powel (Ed). Chapel Hill: University of North Carolina Press.

NAACP requests hospital change. (1966, March 6). *The Daily Times News*, p. 2, 11.

Need of Colored hospital large. (1950, September 12). [Clipping from *The Public Ledger*, an Oxford, NC newspaper]. Granville County Public Library, Oxford, NC.

Negotiated segregation in Salem. (n.d.). Retrieved from: http://www.learnnc.org/lp/editions/nchist-antebellum/5314.

Negro Health Security Company. (1941, March 30). *Asheville Citizen Times*, p. B-3–4.

The Negro Hospital. (1920, November 15). *The Wilmington Star*, p. 4.

Negro hospital opens its doors. (1929, January 15). *The Smithfield Herald*, p. 1.

Negro hospital grows rapidly. (1940, November 16). *Greensboro Record*, n.p.

Negro hospital to open in Greenville, September 1. (1924, August 25). [Clipping from *The Daily Reflector*, a Greenville, NC newspaper]. East Carolina University Library, Greenville, NC.

Negro institution losing money. (1959, November 2). *The Gastonia Gazette*, p. 9.

Negro loses foot. (1912, October 17). *The Statesville Sentinel*, p. 1.

Negro maternity hospital hailed as major step in medical care. (1950, June 19). *The Fayetteville Observer*, p. 1–2.

Negroes of Scotland County meet and pledge loyalty. (1917, July 8). *Wilmington Morning Star*, p. 13.

Negroes to have modern hospital. (1945, July 15). *The Greensboro Daily News*, n.p.

Negroes report on hospital, $833.00. (1926, March 2). *The Smithfield Herald*, p. 8.

New center here in first request for public help (1950, August 11). *The Fayetteville Observer*, p. 2.

New Colored Hospital to open next week. (1943, October 3). *Asheville Citizen*, p. B-8.

New hospital facilities. (1920, January 29). *The Messenger Intelligencer*, p. 1.

A nice donation. (1919, August 5). *Oxford Public Ledger*, p. 5.

North Carolina Board of Health. (1930). One first in which we may take justifiable pride. *The Health Bulletin*, 45(3), 3–8.

North Carolina Board of Medicine. (n.d.). *Doctors*. Retrieved from http://www.ncmedboard.org/timeline.

North Carolina Board of Public Charities. (1906). *Annual report of the Board of Public Charities of North Carolina*. Raleigh, NC: E. M. Uzzell & Company.

North Carolina Board of Public Charities. (1913). *Annual report of the Board of Public Charities of North Carolina*. Raleigh, NC: E. M. Uzzell & Company.

North Carolina Board of Public Charities. (1915). *Annual report of the Board of Public Charities of North Carolina.* Raleigh, NC: E. M. Uzzell & Company.

North Carolina Board of Public Charities. (1917). *Annual report of the Board of Public Charities of North Carolina.* Raleigh, NC: E. M. Uzzell & Company.

North Carolina Hospital and Medical Care Commission. (1945) *To the governor and to the 1945 General Assembly: To the good health of all North Carolina.* Raleigh, NC: The Commission.

North Carolina Hospital and Medical Care Commission. (1947). *Hospital and medical care for all our people: Reports.* Raleigh, NC: The Commission.

North Carolina Nursing History. (2003). Eugene Tranbarger. In *Oral history.* Retrieved from http://nursinghistory.appstate.edu/files/tranbarger-transcript.pdf.

North Carolina Orthopedic Hospital (2016). Retrieved from https://www.stoppingpoints.com/north-carolina/sights.cgi?marker=North+Carolina+Orthopedic+Hospital&cnty=gaston.

The North Carolina State Board of Charities and Public Welfare (1924–1926). *The problem.* Biennial report of The North Carolina State Board of Charities and Public Welfare. Raleigh, NC: Edwards & Broughton Company.

North Carolina State Sanatorium. (1936). *Biennial report of the State Sanatorium.* Retrieved from: http://digital.ncdcr.gov/cdm/compoundobject/collection/p249901coll22/id/163346/rec/1.

Notice of art show. (1886, December 12). *Charlotte Observer,* p. 1.

Nurses October report. (1931, November 6). *Statesville Record,* p. 5.

Oates, J. A. (1950). *The story of Fayetteville and the upper Cape Fear.* Charlotte, NC: The Dowd Press.

The old-timers page. (1954). *Journal of the Old North State Medical Society,* 4(4), 10 & 18.

1,500 persons attend formal opening here for Colored Hospital. (1943, October 22). *Asheville Citizen,* p. A3.

Opening of Sanitarium. (1912, July 23). *The Monroe Journal,* p. 1.

Opening of Shaw Hospital ushers in new era of medical services. (1953, January 20). [Clipping from *The Public Ledger,* an Oxford, NC, newspaper]. Granville County Public Library, Oxford, NC.

Oral History Interview with George Simkins, April 6, 1997. Interview R-0018. Southern Oral History Program Collection (#4007) in the Southern Oral History Program Collection, Southern Historical Collection, Wilson Library, University of North Carolina at Chapel Hill.

Oral History Interview with Mabel Williams, August 20, 1999. Interview K-0266. Southern Oral History Program Collection (#4007) in the Southern Oral History Program Collection, Southern Historical Collection, Wilson Library, University of North Carolina at Chapel Hill.

Pack Memorial Library. (2015). *Students in front of the former Circle Terrace Sanitorium, circa 1922.* Retrieved from https://packlibraryncroom.wordpress.com/students-in-front-of-the-former-circle-terrace-sanitorium-circa-1922/.

Parker, R., & North Carolina. (1990). *Cumberland County: A brief history.* Raleigh, NC: Division of Archives and History, North Carolina Department of Cultural Resources.

Parran, T. (1938). *Shadow of the land: Syphilis the white man's burden.* New York: American Social Hygiene Association.

Peace, S. T. (1956). *"Zeb's Black Baby," Vance County, North Carolina: A short history*. Henderson, NC: Publisher not identified.

Pearson, R. L. (2002). "There are many sick, feeble, and suffering freedmen": The Freedmen's Bureau's health-care activities during Reconstruction in North Carolina, 1865–1868. *North Carolina Historical Review, 79*(2), 141–181.

Phillippe, W. R. (2015). *The pastor's diary: How a conventional conservative became a theological liberal*. Pittsburgh, PA: Author.

Phillips, R. L. (1993). *Medical shoulders during the 19th and 20th centuries in Greensboro, North Carolina*. Greensboro, NC: The Printworks.

Phillips, R. L. (1996). *History of hospitals in Greensboro, North Carolina*. Greensboro, NC: The Printworks.

Piedmont Directory Company. (1907–1952). *Asheville city directories*. Asheville, NC: Piedmont Directory Company.

Piedmont Directory Company. (1920). *Greensboro city directories*. Greensboro, NC: Piedmont Directory Company.

Piedmont Directory Company. (1921). *Greensboro city directories*. Greensboro, NC: Piedmont Directory Company.

A place of their own: The history of Mercy Hospital, Wilson, NC. (1996). Wilson, NC: Community Stories Project.

Pollitt, P. A. and Reese, C. (1999). Jane Renwick Smedburg Wilkes. *American History of Nursing Bulletin, Spring,* 4–6.

Pollitt, P. A., & Reese, C. (2002). Nursing in North Carolina during the Civil War. *Confederate Veteran, 2,* 23–34.

Pollitt, P. A. (2014). *The history of professional nursing in North Carolina 1902–2002*. Durham, NC: Carolina Academic Press.

Pollitt, P. A. (2015). Charlotte Rhone: nurse, welfare worker and entrepreneur. *American Journal of Nursing, 115* (2), 66–70.

Pollitt, P. A., & Leonard, A. (2014). Caring for communities in "The Land of the Sky": Health care institutions and Asheville multiculturalism, 1880s–1920s. *Journal of the North Carolina Association of Historians, 14,* 1–16.

Pollitt, P. A. (2016a). *African American and Cherokee nurses in Appalachia: 1900–1965*. Jefferson, NC: McFarland Press.

Pollitt, P. A. (2016b). Esther McCready, RN: Nursing Advocate for Civil Rights. *OJIN: The Online Journal of Issues in Nursing, 21*(2), 1.

Powell, W. S. (2006). *Wake County*. Retrieved from: http://ncpedia.org/geography/wake.

Pozner, R. (2015, July 20). Asheville's growth began with 19th century TB treatment. *Asheville Citizen-Times*. Retrieved from: http://www.citizen-times.com/story/life/2015/07/20/ashevilles-growth-began-th-century-tb-treatment/30408281/.

Prichard, R. W. (1976). Winston-Salem's Black hospitals prior to 1930. *Journal of the National Medical Association, 68*(3), 246–249.

Pritchett, H. S. (1910). *Introduction: Medical education in the United States and Canada*. New York: The Carnegie Foundation.

Private hospital at North Carolina. (1923, June 30). *New York Age,* p. 2.

Professor Washington. (1905, March 12). *Winston-Salem Journal,* p. 1.

Ptak, J. (2010). *New map: Distribution of slavery in North Carolina, 1860*. Retrieved from: http://longstreet.typepad.com/thesciencebookstore/2010/07/new-map-distribution-of-slavery-in-north-carolina-1860.html.

Public opening of Colored Hospital. (1920, April 30). *The Gastonia Daily Gazette*, p. 1.
Quigless, M. D. (1994). *Looking back: The way things were.* Nashville, NC: C2 Printing and Design.
Ragan, R. A. (2010). *The history of Gastonia and Gaston County, North Carolina: A vision of America at its best.* Charlotte, NC: Loftin & Company.
Ragland, S. (1991, September 1). Jubilee cures need in Black community. *The Henderson Daily Dispatch*, p. D18–20.
Raleigh. (1925, June 20). *New York Age*, p. 9.
Raleigh doctors endorse project. (1917, November 8). *Raleigh News and Observer*, p. 2.
Raleigh hospital marks 25th year. (1948, August 7). *The Pittsburgh Courier*, p. 15.
Raleigh Ku Klux Klan makes gift to St. Agnes. (1922, March 21). *The Raleigh News and Observer*, p. 2.
Raleigh, NC. (1923, October 27). *The New York Age*, p. 5.
Raleigh to have a colored hospital. (1916, January 13). *New York Age*, p. 1.
Rann, E. (1964). The Good Samaritan Hospital of Charlotte, North Carolina. *Journal of the National Medical Association, 56* (3), 223–226.
Rates raised at hospital for Negroes. (1957, August 21). *The Gastonia Gazette*, p. 16.
Rauhauser-Smith, K. (2012). A history of healing. *Winston-Salem Monthly.* Retrieved from: http://www.journalnow.com/winstonsalemmonthly/a-history-of-healing/article_2743c69f-57dc-54ab-b936-75e4d4179c97.html.
Rauhauser-Smith, K. (2015). History-Makers: Simon G. Atkins. *Winston Salem Monthly.* Retrieved from: http://www.journalnow.com/winstonsalemmonthly/history-makers-simon-g-atkins/article_656f0ef2-b7af-11e4-9743-f3a8fbb4e30b.html.
Reed, E. (2008). *Dr. Milton Douglas Quigless, Sr.* Retrieved from: http://www.findagrave.com/cgi-bin/fg.cgi?page=gr&GRid=26885510&ref=acom.
Reese, J. (2014, March 11). Finding Statesville's nurse Daisy. *Statesville Landmark and Record.* Retrieved from: http://www.statesville.com/community/column-finding-statesville-s-nurse-daisy/article_a03cab9a-a868-11e3-b8dd-0017a43b2370.html.
Report from the Colored Hospital. (1888, February 1). *The Charlotte Observer*, p. 4.
Report of the Colored Hospital. (1887, April 19). *The Charlotte Observer*, p. 4.
Report of the Commissioner of Education. (1907). Retrieved from: https://books.google.com/books?id=FMpMAQAAMAAJ&pg=PA1280&lpg=PA1280&dq=Slater+Hospital+Winston+Salem+NC+Hairston&source=bl&ots=D93yuEUWga&sig=y3jtehB0LIDAuPumV3gkp0pwmQU&hl=en&sa=X&ved=0ahUKEwimvqD8r-7MAhWFmx4KHR4qC1kQ6AEIOzAF#v=onepage&q=Slater%20Hospital%20Winston%20Salem%20NC%20Hairston&f=false.
Report to the community. [Booklet]. (1948). Found in the archives of the Episcopal Diocese of Eastern North Carolina, Kinston, NC.
Reports of committees. (1919, September 24). *The Greensboro Daily News*, p. 9.
Reynolds, P. P. (1997). Hospitals and Civil Rights, 1945–1963: The Case of Simkins v. Moses H. Cone Memorial Hospital. *Annals of Internal Medicine, 126* (11), 898–906.
Reynolds, P. P. (2001). *Durham's Lincoln Hospital.* Charleston, SC: Arcadia Press.

Reynolds, P. Preston. (2004). Professional and Hospital DISCRIMINATION and the US Court of Appeals Fourth Circuit 1956–1967. *American Journal of Public Health, 94*(5), 710–720.

Rice, M., & Jones, W. (1994). *Public Policy and the Black Hospital: From Slavery to Segregation to Integration*. Westport, CT: Greenwood Press.

Rives, A. (1922, October 7). Blue Ridge Hospital opened for race by Asheville folks. *The New York Age*, p. 2.

Rosenberg, C. E. (1987). *The care of strangers: The rise of America's hospital system*. New York: Basic Books.

Rotarians endorse St. Agnes. (1922, March 14). *Raleigh News and Observer*, p.10.

A Rotary started hospital for Negroes. (1944). *The Rotarian, 65*(2), 20–21.

Roundtree, T. J. *(2002). Strengthening Ties That Bind: A History of Saint Augustine's College*. Raleigh, NC: St. Augustine's College: Spirit Press.

Rutkow, I. M. (2005). *Bleeding Blue and Gray: Civil War surgery and the evolution of American medicine*. New York: Random House.

Ryan, C. (1964, August 27). Negro hospital is one of few. *The High Point Enterprise*, p. 5.

St. Agnes Hospital. (1926, December 18). *The Raleigh Times*, p. A-8.

St. Agnes Hospital. (1931). *St. Augustine Record. 372*). p. 1.

St. Agnes Hospital. (1932). *St. Augustine Record. 38*(2). p. 2.

St. Agnes Hospital. (1933). *St. Augustine Record. 39*(1). p. 2.

Sale of real estate. (1920, April 9). *Oxford Public Ledger*, p. 7.

Salome Taylor Day proclaimed in Wilmington. (1963, May 8). *The Wilmington Star*, p. 2.

Sammons, V. O. (1990). *Blacks in science and medicine*. New York: Hemisphere Publishing.

Sanitarium for colored people. (1914, June 7). *The Winston-Salem Journal*, p. 7.

Savitt, T. L. (1984). "The Education of Black Physicians at Shaw University, 1882–1918," in J. J. Crow and F. J. Hatley, eds., *Black Americans in North Carolina and the South*. Chapel Hill: University of North Carolina Press.

Savitt, T. L. (1999). Medical history: A medical school for African Americans in 19th century North Carolina. *Department of Medical Humanities Newsletter 2* (2). Retrieved from: http://www.ecu.edu/cs-dhs/medhum/newsletter/v2n2medschool.cfm.

School property given for Colored Hospital building. (1938, March 22). [Clipping from *The Public Ledger*, an Oxford, NC newspaper]. Granville County Public Library, Oxford, NC.

Scruggs, L. A. (1886, April 9). Medical education as a factor in elevation of the colored race. *The African Expositor*, p. 3.

Scruggs, L. A. (1890). *Report to the Raleigh mayor and Board of Alderman*. Retrieved from: https://books.google.com/books?id=uPxOAAAAYAAJ&pg=PA116&lpg=PA116&dq=the+emigrants+we+took+almost+lifeless+from+the+depot+died&source=bl&ots=n7gSABOFAK&sig=z7SBDjYP4i6vR2gffpJI69qPOUQ&hl=en&sa=X&ved=0ahUKEwjEzoGTq83LAhVH6yYKHcOaChsQ6AEIITAA#v=onepage&q=the%20emigrants%20we%20took%20almost%20lifeless%20from%20the%20depot%20died&f=false.

Scruggs, L.A. (1893). *Women of distinction: Remarkable in works and invincible in character*. Raleigh: L.A. Scruggs.

Scruggs, L. A. (1897). Pickford Sanitarium. *The Southern Sanitarian 1*(4), 1. Retrieved from http://docsouth.unc.edu/nc/scruggs/scruggs.html.

Scruggs, L. A. (1900). Our immediate needs. *The Southern Sanitarium* 3(9), 18–19.
Scruggs, L. A. (1901). Some interesting reflections upon the physical life of a Negro. *The Southern Sanitarium* 4(11), 6, 17 & 18.
Scruggs, L. A. (1901). An appeal to you. *The Southern Sanitarium* 1(6), 9.
Sebastian, S. P. (1930). The L. Richardson Memorial Hospital. *Journal of the National Medical Association, 22*(3), 142–144.
Several hospitals preceded current Carolina East (2013, April 21). *The Sun Journal*, p. 1. Retrieved from: http://www.newbernsj.com/article/20130421/News/304219962.
Shaw celebrates founder Dr. Henry Martin Tupper's birthday. (2014, April 11). Retrieved from: http://www.shawu.edu/Shaw_Celebrates_Founder_Dr_Henry_Martin_Tupper_s_Birthday.aspx.
Shaw Hospital opens for patients Jan. 31. (1953, January 30). [Clipping from *The Public Ledger*, an Oxford, NC newspaper]. Granville County Public Library, Oxford, NC.
Shaw Hospital to be shown next Tuesday. (1952, November 25). [Clipping from *The Public Ledger*, an Oxford, NC newspaper]. Granville County Public Library, Oxford, NC.
Shepard, C. H. (1930). The Lincoln Hospital. *Journal of the National Medical Association 22*(3), 139–140.
Shinn, J. (1962, March 4). Unidentified man tears signs of Negro pickets at hospital. *The Charlotte Observer*, p. 1
Shower of linens and money. (1926). *Women's Missionary Magazine 40*(3), 791.
Shrandy, G. F., & Stedman, T. L. (1899). Some of the problems of the alienist. *Medical Records* 55, 773–778.
Shuford, P. S. (1975). Oral history interview of Dr. Polly Shuford. Retrieved from http://toto.lib.unca.edu/findingaids/oralhistory/SHRC/shuford_polly.htmSilberman, P. (2010). History of health care policy making in North Carolina. Retrieved from: https://iei.ncsu.edu/wp-content/uploads/2013/02/Silberman-History-of-Health.pdf.
Silver and china donated to the Negro hospital from the Women's Civic Club. (1954, October 20). [Clipping from *The Gastonia Gazette*, a Gastonia, NC newspaper]. Gaston County Public Library, Gastonia, NC.
Simkins v. M. H. Cone Hospital, 323 F.2d 959 (1963).
Sisters of Charity conduct fine Greensboro hospital. (1931, September 26). *The Bulletin of the Catholic Layman's Association of Georgia*, p. 4.
Slater Hospital. (1909, April 30). *The Western Sentinel*, p. 1.
Slater Hospital. (2016). Retrieved from: http://www.digitalforsyth.org/photos/stories/slater-hospital.
Slater Hospital closed. (1910, November 5). *Winston-Salem Journal*, p. 1.
Slater Normal School (1903, May 15). *Winston-Salem Journal*, p. 1.
Smith, S. L. (1995). *Sick and tired of being sick and tired: Black women's health activism in America, 1890–1950*. Philadelphia: University of Pennsylvania Press.
Society and personal. (1913). *Journal of the National Medical Association, 5*(4), p. 278.
Spencer, M. B. (1919, April 4). A colored woman's plea for a hospital. *The Public Ledger*, p. 1.

Srikanth, S. (2016). Edgecombe County. Retrieved from: http://northcarolina history.org/encyclopedia/edgecombe-county-1741/.
Starr, P. (1982). *The social transformation of American medicine*. New York: Basic Books.
State Archives of North Carolina. (2016). McCauley Private Hospital. Retrieved from: https://www.flickr.com/photos/north-carolina-state-archives/247721 99726.
Steelman, B. (2011). Who was Salome Taylor? Retrieved from: http://www.myreporter.com/2011/02/who-was-salome-taylor/.
Steuart W. M. (1922). *Mortality statistics 1920, twenty-first annual report*. Washington, D.C.: U.S. Government Printing Office.
Substantial aid for sanitarium. (1898, July 7). *The Morning Post*, p. 5.
Successful entertainment. (1903, July 7). *The Winston-Salem Journal*, p. 1.
Superintendent's Report for the Year of 1884. (1884). Retrieved from: http://docsouth.unc.edu/nc/eastern84/eastern84.html.
Susie Cheatham Hospital. (1949, October 18). *The Gastonia Gazette*, p. 1.
Tag day set for Slater Hospital. (1909, August 24). *The Western Sentinel*, p. 2.
Tan seats on hospital board asked. (1965, January 2). *The Afro American*, p. 27.
This week in Lumberton. (1910, July 3). *The Wilmington Morning Star*, p. 3.
Thomas, K. K. (1997). Oral History Interview with Andrew Best, April 19, 1997. Interview R-0011. Southern Oral History Program Collection (#4007). Retrieved from: http://docsouth.unc.edu/sohp/R-0011/R-0011.html.
Thomas, K. K. (2006). The Hill-Burton Act and civil rights: Expanding hospital care for Black southerners, 1939–1960. *The Journal of Southern History*, 72(4), 823–870.
Thomas, K. K. (2011). *Deluxe Jim Crow: Civil rights and American health policy, 1935–1954*. Athens: University of Georgia Press.
Thornton, P. (2007). Granville history. In. Retrieved from: http://www.granvillemuseumnc.org/granville.htmlhttp://www.granvillemuseumnc.org/granville.html.
3 race students enter U. of N.C. (1951, June 16). *The Pittsburgh Courier*, p. 1.
Training colored youth. (1895, January 11). *The Charlotte Observer*, p. 5.
Union County Medical Society Auxiliary. (1968). *Union County men of medicine*. Monroe, NC: Union County Medical Society Auxiliary.
The Union Hospital. (1894, April 15). *The Charlotte Observer*, p. 6.
Ushers Union gives oxygen tent to hospital. (1954, August 12). [Clipping from *The Gastonia Gazette*, a Gastonia, NC newspaper]. Gaston County Public Library, Gastonia, NC.
U.S. Census Bureau (1860, 1880, 1890, 1900, 1910, 1920, 2010). Retrieved from http://docsouth.unc.edu/classroom/lessonplans/gtts/city_directory.html.
Valentine, P. M. (2002). *The rise of a southern town, Wilson, NC 1840–1920*. Baltimore, MD: Gateway Press, Inc.
Walden, H. N. (1964). *History of Union County*. Charlotte, NC: Heritage Printers, Inc.
Ward, T. J. (2003). *Black physicians in the Jim Crow south*. Fayetteville: University of Arkansas Press.
Waters, D. J. (2012). *Life beneath the veneer: The Black community in Asheville, North Carolina from 1793 to 1900*. (Unpublished doctoral dissertation). University of North Carolina, Chapel Hill, NC.

Watson, A. D. (1987). *A history of New Bern and Craven County*. New Bern, NC: Tryon Palace Commission.
Watson, A. D. (1979). *Edgecombe County, a brief history*. Raleigh, NC: North Carolina Dept. of Cultural Resources, Division of Archives and History.
Watts, C. D., & Scott, F. W. (1965). Lincoln Hospital of Durham, North Carolina. *Journal of the National Medical Association, 57*(2), 177–185.
Way, J. H., & McBrayer, L. B. (1928). *Medical colleges in North Carolina*. Raleigh, Authors.
A well-deserved honor. (1952, April 5). *The Carolina Times*, p. 2.
Whitted, J. A. (1908). *A History of the Negro Baptists of North Carolina*. Raleigh, NC: Edwards & Broughton Printing Company.
Wicker, E. (2013). *Voices: Lincoln Hospital School of Nursing*. Fuquay-Varina, NC: Jones Booker Publishing.
Widely known Negro nurse Mrs. Dorothy Crawford died here. (1947, November 29). *The Gastonia Gazette*, p. 10.
Wilkerson, I. O. (1992). History of the North Carolina Medical Care Commission. *North Carolina Medical Journal 53*(1), 42–48.
Wilkes, F. (1939). Good Samaritan Hospital. *Southern Hospital 7*(12), 9–10.
Williams, A. C. (1994). *Rex Hospital: A centennial celebration*. Raleigh, NC: Rex Hospital.
Williams, B. (1950, March 28). Additions and improvements to the Gaston County Colored Hospital will add greatly to its efficiency. [Clipping from *The Gastonia Gazette*, a Gastonia, NC newspaper]. Gaston County Public Library, Gastonia, NC.
Williams, D. (2011, February 18). *U.S. Colored Troops/Granville County*. Retrieved from http://www.ncgenweb.us/ncgranville/military/usctgran.htmhttp://www.ncgenweb.us/ncgle/military/usct-gran.htm.
Williams, W. C. (2001). *PMCH: A tradition of excellence*. Raleigh, NC: Barefoot Press.
Wilmington, NC. (1924, May 10). *The Pittsburgh Courier*, p. 10.
Womble, J. (2002, February 24). Fayetteville's Perry was a medical pioneer. *The Fayetteville Observer*. Retrieved from: http://www.fayobserver.com/living/fayetteville-s-perry-was-a-medical-pioneer/article_31d9d58c-7284-5980-9999-f8c71090c0a4.html.
Women's and children's division. (1922, November 17). *The Messenger-Intelligencer*, p. 6.
Woodbury, R. H. (n.d.). *Blue Ridge Hospital* [Brochure]. Heritage of Black Highlanders Collection, D. H. Ramsey Library, University of North Carolina Asheville.
Woodward, C. V. (1974). *The strange career of Jim Crow*. New York: Oxford University Press.
Wright, M. (2006). Laurinburg Institute. Retrieved from http://ncpedia.org/laurinburg-normal-and-industrial-in.
Yenser, T. (1942). McCauley, L. E. In *Who's who in Colored America*. (Vol. 6. pp. 335–336). New York: Author.
Yourd, S. (1911). The Jubilee Hospital, Henderson, NC. *The Women's Missionary Magazine, 25*(2), 39–40.
Zogry, K. J. (2008). The house that Dr. Pope built: Race, politics, memory and the early struggle for civil rights in North Carolina. (Unpublished doctoral dissertation). University of North Carolina, Chapel Hill, NC.

Index

Abbot, Dr. M.S.G. 40
Adams, Dinah Ada, RN 89
Adams, Doris, RN 146
Adams, Eva Johnson, RN 102, 103, 105, 107
Alexander, Carrie L., RN 103
Allen, Gertrude, RN 103
Allen, Dr. Hobart Theodor 82
Alston, Sadie, RN 141
Anderson, Edith, RN 144, 145
Armstrong, Marchusa, RN 146
The Asheville Colored Hospital 11, 98–100, 171
Ashford, Dr. 145
Atkins, Simon Green 76–77
Avant, Dr. Frank 16, 129–130
Avery, Dr. Parnell 102

Barnes, Dr. B.O. 92
Barnette, Magnolia B., RN 103
Baskerville, Lucinda, LPN 121
Baxter, Dr. John Earl 16, 102
Beckford, Dr. Samuel McDonald 102
Berber, Lillie Forte, RN 115
Best, Dr. Andrew 138
Betsch, Cleo, RN 103
Bigelow Hospital 16, 140–142, 152, 170, 173
Blair, Eugenia, LPN 127
Blue Ridge Hospital and school of nursing 11, 15, 16, 95–99, 170, 173
Bobbitt, Irene, LPN 119, 121
Bowens, Dr. 130
Boyd, Hazel Neely, RN 127
Bradsher, Dr. J.S. 121
Brevard, Dr. R.J. 58
Brinson, Dorothy 53
Broadfoot, Carrie Early, RN 165–167
Broadhurst, RN 119, 121
Broughton, Gov. Melvin 27

Broughton Hospital 162, 164
Brown, Dr. A.J. 78
Brown v. Board of Education Supreme Court case 31, 33
Bryant, Dr. David 131
Bryant, Dr. Reuben 15, 96, 99
Buchanan, Mrs. Annie Robinson, RN 63
Bugg, Dr. James, 40
Burch, Georgiana, RN 155
Burnett, Dr. Foster 130, 131

Caldwell, Dr. D.E. 15, 63
Calloway, Nellie R. RN, 113
Carpenter, Mary, RN 103
Carrington, Dr. S.M. 119, 121
Carter, Patty, RN 72
Carter, Dr. W. Perry 126
Cartwright, Dr. Samuel 22
Charlotte Home and Hospital 13, 56, 60
Cheatham, Henry 118–119
Cherry Hospital (North Carolina Colored Insane Asylum) 8, 1, 14, 160–164
Chestnut, Dr. 130
Christmas, Dr. Mathew D. 16
Circle Terrace Sanatorium 15, 93–95, 170, 173
Civil Rights Act of 1964 11, 32–34, 85, 87, 92, 101, 116, 121, 134, 147, 157, 164, 165, 168, 170, 171
Civil War era hospitals 7–8
Clay, Dr. E.L. 121
Cleland, Dr. William A. 74
Coe, Mabel, RN 131
Collins, Geneva Sitrena RN 95
Colored Branch, Davis Hospital, Statesville, North Carolina 138–140, 173

Index

Colored/Union Hospital 15, 57–60
Colson, Dr. Joseph 121
Colvert, Henrietta, RN 89
Community Hospital 11, 14, 16, 128–134
Corbett, Katie, RN 113
Cordice, Dr. John Walter Vincent 111
Cordice Sanitarium 11, 14, 111
Cotton, Rev. John Adams 102, 104
Cowan, Annie Mae, RN 89
Cowan, Dr. J.E. 89 92
Crawford, Dorothy Hemphill, RN 77
Culpepper, Geneva H., RN 141
Cunningham, Lois Rice, RN 95

Daniel, Dr. Sam 121
Darst, Bishop Robert 144
Davis, Elizabeth Viola, RN 103
Davis, Fred 90–91
Davis, Mrs. V.C. 146
Dellinger, Mrs. J.E. 115
Diggs, Dr. Edward O. 38
Dissoway, Dr. Lula 146
Dix Hill Sanitarium 7
Dr. Eaton's Sanitorium 152
Dr. Erwin's Hospital 11, 16, 125–127
Dr. Hargrave's Hospital 11, 15, 87, 90
Donnell, Inez, RN 113
Duffey, Dr. 145
Duke, Benjamin 73
Duke, James B. 25, 167–168
Duke, Washington 12, 70, 172
The Duke Endowment 25–27, 51, 63, 74, 82, 90, 99, 104–105, 115, 120, 127, 128, 133, 144–145, 170, 174
Duke Pavilion, Negro Division State Orthopedic Hospital 168
DuPont Maud Beulah, RN 95

Eaton, Dr. Chester A. 16, 151
Eaton, Dr. Hubert 4, 18, 31, 83, 130, 134, 152, 171
Eisenhower, Dwight 18
Elliott, Dr. J.C. 121
Elliott. Mary, RN 166
English, Dr. W.T. 21
Enloe, Mary Montgomery, RN 77h
Erwin, Dr. Herbert Jones 16, 125
Exon, Roxanna, RN 90

Faison, Dr. J.W. 63
Faison, Dr. William 163
Fisher, Dr. 145
Fitzgerald, Sallie, RN 113

Flexner Report 43–46
Fort Bragg, Fayetteville, North Carolina 17, 144, 152–154
Frances, Inez Dudley, RN 146
Freedman's Bureau era Hospitals in North Carolina 8–9
Freedman's Hospital, Washington, D.C. 43
Freeman, Oliver Nestus 88, 90
Furlonge, Dr. Charles William 16, 122–124
Furlonge Hosptial 16, 121–124

Gallego, Dr. Louis N. 96
Gaston County Colored Hospital 25, 126–128, 171
Glenn, Dr. Charles 126
Good Samaritan Hospital 12, 13, 15, 19, 25, 27, 29, 59, 60–65, 125, 149, 155, 169, 172
Good Shepherd Hospital 12, 16, 25, 142–147, 171, 174
Grady, Dr. L.V. 90
Grandy, Augusta I., RN 119
Gray, Dr. Samuel Jones 31, 133
Green, A.B. 74
Green, Frances, RN 92
Green, Dr. James P. 102
Green, Dr. Paul S. 102
Green, Dr. William E. 102
Groves, Anna, nurse 48

Hacker, Joan, RN 103
Hairston, Lula C. RN 77
Hall, Alice 53
Hall, Dr. H. Humphrey 15, 77
Hargrave, Dr. Frank Settle 15, 77, 87–88, 89, 90, 92, 103
Hargrave, Mary, RN 103
Hawkins, O.W. 4
Hawkins, Dr. Reginald 65, 170
Heard, Estelle Virginia, LPN 121
Hennie, Rebecca, RN 119, 145
Henry, Dr. John 81
Henry, Mae, RN 155
Hines, William 90
Hirshinger, Mrs. 57, 59
Hobbs, Versie 53
Holt, Dr. John P. 16, 100
Holt, Dr. John Walker 16, 96
Hopkins, Frances, RN 137–138
Hospital Survey and Construction Act/Hill-Burton Act 29–30
Howard University 46, 111
Hunt, Hettie Jim 103
Hunter, A.B. 47, 78–79

Index

Hunter, Dr. 141
Hunter, Sarah 47, 78–79

Jackson, Charlotte, RN 63
Jackson, Della Raney, RN 17, 75
Jackson, Dr. Nathaniel Edward 16, 141, 152
James, Helen, RN 92
James A. Walker Memorial Hospital, Wilmington, North Carolina 14, 18, 31, 129, 130, 134, 171
Jeflers, Madge, RN 53
Johnson, Cora, RN 126
Johnson, Robert 57, 144
Johnson, Susan, RN 113
Jones, Fred 90–91
Jones, Dr. John W. 15, 77
Jones, Luvenia, RN 53
Jordan, Dr. J.C. 83
Jubilee Hospital, Henderson, North Carolina 16 101–107, 172

Kafer, Dr. 145
Kate B. Reynolds Memorial Hospital 4, 12, 16, 19, 31, 43, 73, 81–86, 174
Kay, Dr. John Walcott 16, 130, 131
King, Georgia C. RN 131
Ku Klux Klan 49

L. Richardson Memorial Hospital 12, 13, 19, 25, 27, 29, 30, 43, 114–117, 170, 171, 174
Latta, Julia, RN 72
Lawrence, Matilda, RN 103
Leary-Perry Hospital, Fayetteville, North Carolina 11, 16, 150–154, 171, 174
Lentz, George 84
Leonard, Judson 38
Leonard Hospital and Medical School, Raleigh, North Carolina 37–47
Lincoln, Mrs. O.H., RN 154
Lincoln Hospital, Durham, North Carolina 4, 12, 15, 16 43, 70–76, 170, 172
Little, Rubina, nursing student 64
Lofton, Helen, RN 130
Long, Lula, RN 95
Long, Dr. Wesley 110

Malloy, Dr. H.D. 83
Mann, Dr. 145
Marshall, Carrie, nurse 109
Martin, Dr. 145
Massey, Dr. John Sherman 15, 108–110
May, Jeanette, RN 96

Mayo, Salz 28
McCauley, Dr. Llewyn 38, 52–55
McCauley Private Hospital, Raleigh, North Carolina 11, 19, 19, 49, 52–56, 170, 173
McClain, Celeste, RN 92
McCloud, Dr. Willard 81
McDuffie, Emanuel Montee 141
McKeown 1
McKinley, Marie, LPN 127
McNeil, Bertha, RN 141
McWrath, Daisy, RN 126
Medicaid 11, 33–34, 75, 85, 92, 117, 138, 154, 157
Medicare 11, 33–34, 75, 85, 92, 117, 121, 138, 154, 157
Meharry Medical School, Nashville, Tennessee 44
Mercy Hospital, Charlotte, North Carolina 59
Mercy Hospital, Hamlet, North Carolina 152, 155
Mercy Hospital, Wilson, North Carolina 16, 87, 90–92, 173, 174
Metz, Flossie, RN 95, 96
Miller, Edna, RN 100
Miller, Dr. Lee Otis 96, 97
Mills, Dr. Joseph Napolean 16
Mission Hospital, Asheville, North Carolina 14, 96, 97, 101
Missouri ex rel, Gaines v. Canada Supreme Court case 31
Mitchner, Dr. W.A 89, 92
Monroe, Dr. John 107
Moore, Dr. Aaron McDuffie 15, 70, 72, 169
Moore, Laura, RN 146
Moore, Mary A. RN 123
Moore, Rev. W.H. 130
Morehead, Mrs. Eliza, RN 57
Moses H. Cone Memorial Hospital, Greensboro, North Carolina 110, 116
Mount Tirzah Hospital, Wilmington, North Carolina 7
Mumford, Dr. 145

National Medical Association 55, 57, 124, 136
Noblin, Dr. R.L., 119
North Carolina Board of Dental Examiners 30
North Carolina Board of Medicine and Medical Examiners 30, 40
North Carolina Board of Nursing Examiners 30

North Carolina Health Bulletin 23
North Carolina Medical Care Commission 27–28
North Carolina Medical Society 31, 124, 151, 171
North Carolina Mental Health Council 30
North Carolina Nurse Association 30
North Carolina State Board of Charities and Public Welfare 21, 78, 80
North Carolina State Board of Health 30, 66, 74
North Carolina State Board of Nursing 19, 54, 63, 73, 84, 114, 133
North Carolina State Orthopedic Hospital—Negro Division 13, 160, 167–168, 170, 173
North Carolina State Sanitarium—Negro Division 13, 19, 94, 164–167
Northern, Lillian, RN 81
Norwood Dr. Ballard 121

O'Donoghue, Dr. Dennis 62
Old North State Medical Society 54, 55, 87, 124, 130, 169, 171
Oteen Military/Veteran's Administration Hospital, Asheville, North Carolina 17

Parran, Thomas 21
Parris, Dr. 130
Patterson, A. Elizabeth, RN 141
Pearson, Conrad 32
Peoples, Nina E. RN 79
Perry, Dr. Golan S. 53
Perry, Dr. John S. 152
Perry, Dr. Mathew Leary 16, 152–153
Person, Ora Lee, RN 121
Phillip, M.L., RN 146
Pickford Sanitarium 4, 11, 15, 65–70, 170, 172
Plessy v. Ferguson Supreme Court Case 17, 20, 159, 169
Plummer, Ida Mae, RN 103
Pope, Dr. M.T. 15, 40, 63, 169
Powell, Adam Clayton 18
Powell, Dr. Simon 16
Pressley, Dr. H.W. 63
Prince, Dr. A.T. 40

Quality Hill Sanatorium 11, 15, 107–110, 173
Quick, Dr. C. Mason 151
Quigless, Helen 149
Quigless, Dr. Milton Douglas 4, 148–150

Quigless, Dr. Milton Douglas, Jr. 150
Quigless Clinic 4, 11, 147–150, 171, 174

Rabb, Mattie, RN 126
Raleigh Academy of Medicine 45
Randolph, Emma Lee RN 75
Randolph, Dr. Robert 74
Ray, Dr. Alexander Hamilton 16, 81
Ray's Hospital 11, 16, 81, 170, 173
Redding, Claretta, nurse 166
Reed, Daisy, RN 102
Reid, Mrs J., RN 114
Reid, J.D. 88
Rex Hospital 14, 34, 47, 54
Reynolds, R.J. 12, 32, 76, 77, 85, 172
Reynolds, William Neal 16, 82–83, 174
Reynolds Memorial Hospital, Winston-Salem, North Carolina 85
Richardson, Lunsford 114
Richardson, Madeline, RN 53
Richardson, Mary Lynn 12, 114
River, Dr. Tomas Monte 135–136
Rivera Clinic 11, 135–136, 170, 173
Roane, Dr. Daniel 31, 133, 171
Roberts, Dr. Peter F. 53
Robertson, Lillian, RN 109
Robinson, Carrie, RN 94
Robinson, Daisy Connor, RN 139–140, 170, 173
Robinson, Dr. Joseph 141
Rosenwald Fund 26–27, 144, 174

St. Agnes Hospital and School of Nursing 4, 112, 14, 19, 25, 27, 29 38, 43, 47–55, 67, 72, 73, 78, 79, 80, 87, 89, 90, 119, 122, 131, 135, 166, 170, 172
St. Augustine College/University 37, 38, 46–48, 51, 52, 67, 76
St. Frances Hospital, Greenville, North Carolina 136–138, 170, 173
St. Leo's Hospital 14, 110
Sanitarium, Fayetteville, North Carolina 16
Scott, F.W. 75
Scruggs, Dr. L.A. 14 40, 65–70, 169, 170
Sears, Mattie, RN 96
Sebastian, Dr. Simon Powell 111, 112, 113, 114, 115
Segregated hospital beds by county 28
Shaw, Parnell, RN 146
Shaw Memorial Hospital 11, 121, 171, 174
Shaw University 12, 36, 37, 38, 45, 47, 48, 67, 122

Index

Shepard, Dr. Charles H. 15, 72
Sheppard, Elizabeth Davis, RN 121
Shuford, Dr. Mary "Polly" 11, 97, 98, 174
Shuford Clinic 11, 97, 98, 99, 171, 174
Simkins, George 31, 32, 116, 171
Simkins v. Moses H. Cone Memorial Hospital 31, 32, 33, 87, 92, 116, 121, 134, 147, 157, 165, 168
Skinner, Mrs. M.H., RN 146
Slater Hospital 4, 12, 14, 15 19, 76–80, 87, 170, 172
Sloan, Dr. James M. 126
Smith, Annie L., RN 119
Smith, Flora, RN 123
Smith, Maggie Esther, RN 103
The Southern Sanitarian 68–69
Spellman, T. Beatrice 109
Spencer, Martha, RN 117
Spring, Eva, RN 127
Sternberger Bertha 114
Stewart, Dr. Charles Constantine 112–113
Stewart, Dr. H.D. 107
Strudwick, Dr. William C. 16
Sullivan, Dr. 92
Susie Cheatham Hospital 11, 25, 29, 118–121, 171, 173

Tate, Idell RN 96
Taylor, Dancy 53
Taylor, Elina 53
Taylor, Mary, RN 113
Taylor, Dr. R.W. 121
Taylor, Salome, RN 131, 133
Taylor, Dr. W.L. 119, 121
Thomas, Dr. W.N. 119, 121
Thompson, Dr. 96
Thorton, F.J. 53
Toney, Dr. Ellis E. 119, 121
Torrence, Dr. William Green 93
Torrence Hospital 11, 14, 93, 170, 172
Trinity Hospital 11, 16, 112
Trollinger, Virginia, RN 127
Truman, Harry 18
Tupper, Henry and Sarah 38
Tuskegee Institute 78, 135, 141
Tuskegee Study 22
Twin Cities Medical Society 81–82

Union County Medical Society 108
United States Department of Health, Education and Welfare 34, 65
United States Public Health Service 7, 22, 113
University of North Carolina School of Medicine 18, 38

Vass, Dr. Rufus Samuel 53
Vault, Dr. Mintauts 163
Venable, Dr. Robert
Vick, S.H. 88

Wadsworth, Dr. 145
Wake County Memorial Hospital 54
Walker, Dr. John Wakefield 15, 93–94, 96
Warren, Dr. Stanford Lee 15, 72
Watkins, Dr. G. Sam 119
Watson, R.P. 90
Watts Hospital 14, 71, 75–76, 170
Webb, Charles 98
Whitted, Bessie, RN 92
Whittington, Dr. J.B. 83
Wilkes, Mrs. Jane, nurse 58–62
Williams, Daniel Hale 35
Williams, Dr. J.T. 15, 40, 58, 62
Williamson, Dr. John C. 16, 80
Williamson Sanitarium 11, 16 80–81, 170, 173
Williston, Dr. Thomas H. 126
Wills, Kathleen, RN 95
Wilson, Helen, RN 92
Wilson, Nettie, RN 75
Wilson Colored Hospital 90, 171, 174
Wilson Hospital 11
Wilson Hospital and Tubercular Home 87–89, 92, 170
Winfield, Anna B., RN 53
Winston, Annie L. RN 121
Woodard, Dr. C.A. 90
Woodbury, Ruby, RN 95–96
Woods, Sadie RN 96
Wooten, Mrs. Henry 154
World War I 17, 22, 135, 152, 155, 166
World War II 17, 23, 27, 29, 43, 54, 74, 86, 90, 105, 110, 133, 134, 136, 149, 152, 164
Wortham, Effie, RN 48
Wright, Dr. Enos Shepherd 73, 82

www.ingramcontent.com/pod-product-compliance
Ingram Content Group UK Ltd.
Pitfield, Milton Keynes, MK11 3LW, UK
UKHW042005140426
5217IPUK00015B/989